T0263942

Obesity Management in Primary Care

Editor

MARK B. STEPHENS

PRIMARY CARE:
CLINICS IN OFFICE PRACTICE

www.primarycare.theclinics.com

Consulting Editor
JOEL J. HEIDELBAUGH

March 2016 • Volume 43 • Number 1

ELSEVIER

1600 John F. Kennedy Boulevard • Suite 1800 • Philadelphia, Pennsylvania, 19103-2899

http://www.theclinics.com

PRIMARY CARE: CLINICS IN OFFICE PRACTICE Volume 43, Number 1
March 2016 ISSN 0095-4543, ISBN-13: 978-0-323-41659-7

Editor: Jessica McCool
Developmental Editor: Colleen Viola

Primary Care: Clinics in Office Practice (ISSN: 0095–4543) is published quarterly by Elsevier Inc., 360 Park Avenue South, New York, NY 10010-1710. Months of issue are March, June, September, and December. Periodicals postage paid at New York, NY and additional mailing offices. Subscription prices are $225.00 per year (US individuals), $434.00 (US institutions), $100.00 (US students), $275.00 (Canadian individuals), $491.00 (Canadian institutions), $175.00 (Canadian students), $345.00 (international individuals), $491.00 (international institutions), and $175.00 (international students). Foreign air speed delivery is included in all *Clinics* subscription prices. All prices are subject to change without notice. POSTMASTER: Send address changes to *Primary Care: Clinics in Office Practice*, Elsevier Periodicals Customer Service, 11830 Westline Industrial Drive, St. Louis, MO 63146. Customer Service Health Sciences Division, Subscription Customer Service, 3251 Riverport Lane, Maryland Heights, MO 63043. **Customer Service: 1-800-654-2452 (U.S. and Canada); 314-447-8871 (outside U.S. and Canada). Fax: 314-447-8029. E-mail: journalscustomerservice-usa@elsevier.com (for print support); journalsonlinesupport-usa@elsevier.com (for online support).**

Reprints. For copies of 100 or more, of articles in this publication, please contact the Commercial Reprints Department, Elsevier Inc., 360 Park Avenue South, New York, NY 10010-1710. Tel. 212-633-3874; Fax: 212-633-3820; E-mail: reprints@elsevier.com.

Primary Care: Clinics in Office Practice is covered in *MEDLINE/PubMed (Index Medicus)* and *EMBASE/Excerpta Medica, Current Contents/Clinical Medicine,* and *ISI/BIOMED.*

Contributors

CONSULTING EDITOR

JOEL J. HEIDELBAUGH, MD, FAAFP, FACG
Clinical Professor, Departments of Family Medicine and Urology; Clerkship Director, Department of Family Medicine, University of Michigan Medical School, Ann Arbor, Michigan; Ypsilanti Health Center, Ypsilanti, Michigan

EDITOR

MARK B. STEPHENS, MD, MS, FAAFP, CAPT, MC, USN
Professor and Chair, Department of Family Medicine, Uniformed Services University, Bethesda, Maryland

AUTHORS

KEVIN M. BERNSTEIN, MD, MMS
Lieutenant Commander, Medical Corps, United States Navy; Staff Family Physician, Fleet Surgical Team SEVEN, Okinawa, Japan

KENDALL M. CAMPBELL, MD
Associate Professor and Co-director, Department of Family Medicine and Rural Health, The Center for Underrepresented Minorities in Academic Medicine, Florida State University College of Medicine, Tallahassee, Florida

OMNI CASSIDY, MS
Doctoral Candidate, Department of Medical and Clinical Psychology, Uniformed Services University of the Health Sciences, Bethesda, Maryland

MARC DIFAZIO, MD
Medical Director of the Montgomery County Outpatient Center, Medical Director of Ambulatory Neurology, Department of Neurology, Children's National Health System, Rockville, Maryland

DANIELLE SYMONS DOWNS, PhD
Professor of Kinesiology and Obstetrics & Gynecology, Director, Exercise Psychology Laboratory, Department of Kinesiology, College of Health and Human Development, Pennsylvania State University, University Park, Pennsylvania

JILL EMERICK, MD
Assistant Professor, Department of Pediatrics, USUHS, Bethesda, Maryland

JEFF HUTCHINSON, MD, FAAP
Assistant Professor, Department of Pediatrics, USUHS, Bethesda, Maryland

JESSICA LYNN JONES, MD, MSPH
Assistant Professor, Division of Public Health, Department of Family and Preventive Medicine, University of Utah, Salt Lake City, Utah

REGINA M. JULIAN, MHA, MBA, FACHE
Chief, Primary Care (Patient Centered Medical Home), Clinical Support Division, Defense Health Agency, Falls Church, Virginia

VIRGINIA B. KALISH, MD
Family Medicine Faculty, National Capital Consortium Family Medicine Residency, Fort Belvoir Community Hospital, Fort Belvoir, Virginia

CLAIRE P. KELLEY, PsyD
Postdoctoral Fellow, Department of Medical and Clinical Psychology, Uniformed Services University of the Health Sciences, Bethesda, Maryland

ELEANOR R. MACKEY, PhD
Assistant Professor, Department of Psychology and Behavioral Health, Children's National Health System, Washington, DC

DEBRA A. MANNING, MD, MBA, FAAFP
Commander, Medical Corps, United States Navy; Director, Medical Home Port, Bureau of Medicine and Surgery, Falls Church, Virginia

ALEXANDRA OLSON, BA
Clinical Research Coordinator, Children's National Health System, Center for Translational Science, Washington, DC

NATASHA PYZOCHA, DO
Department of Family Medicine, Madigan Army Medical Center, Fort Lewis, Washington

SCOTT T. REHRIG Jr, MD, COL, MC
Clinical Associate Professor of Surgery, Uniformed Services University of the Health Sciences, Bethesda, Maryland

JOSÉ E. RODRÍGUEZ, MD
Associate Professor and Co-director, Department of Family Medicine and Rural Health, The Center for Underrepresented Minorities in Academic Medicine, Florida State University College of Medicine, Tallahassee, Florida

HARSHITA SAXENA, MD
Assistant Professor, Department of Pediatrics, USUHS, Bethesda, Maryland

GEENA SBROCCO, MS, RD
Registered Dietician, Loyola University, Chicago, Illinois; Lincoln Park Care Center, Lincoln Park, New Jersey

TRACY SBROCCO, PhD
Professor; Director, Department of Medical and Clinical Psychology, Uniformed Services University of the Health Sciences, Bethesda, Maryland

JULIE SCHWARTZ, MS, RDN, CSSD, LD
Health Promotion Dietitian, Department of Defense, MacDill Air Force Base, Tampa, Florida

KRISTY BREUHL SMITH, MD
Assistant Professor, Department of Community Health and Family Medicine, Assistant Professor, University of Florida, Gainesville, Florida

MICHAEL SETH SMITH, MD, CAQ-SM, PharmD
Assistant Professor, Department of Orthopedics and Rehabilitation, Assistant Professor, University of Florida, Gainesville, Florida

ELENA A. SPIEKER, PhD
Department of Family Medicine, Madigan Army Medical Center, Fort Lewis, Washington; Department of Medical and Clinical Psychology, Uniformed Services University of the Health Sciences, Bethesda, Maryland

DAVID SUNDWALL, MD
Professor, Division of Public Health, Department of Family and Preventive Medicine, University of Utah, Salt Lake City, Utah

MESHIA Q. WALEH, MD
Assistant Professor, Department of Family and Preventive Medicine, University of South Carolina School of Medicine, Columbia, South Carolina

Contents

> The National Health and Nutrition Examination Survey from the Centers for Disease Control and Prevention reports a steady increase in obesity over the last 30 years. The greatest increase was seen in 15 to 19 year olds, whose obesity prevalence almost doubled from 10.5% to 19.4%. The solution to pediatric obesity requires a multidisciplinary approach addressing cultural norms, technologic advances, and family engagement. Future treatment strategies to combat the obesity epidemic will have to extend beyond the health care provider's office. Behavior modification remains the key component to pediatric obesity prevention and treatment.

> Obesity, defined as a body mass index (BMI) of 30 or higher in adults and BMI in the 95th percentile or higher for children, is epidemic in the United States. The predominant culture of caloric excess and sedentary behaviors contributes to this problem. Obesity increases the risk of many chronic diseases and premature death. The broad response to this costly disease includes efforts from medical providers, local and federal governments, and nongovernmental agencies. Although obesity can be addressed on an individual basis, it is largely recognized as a public health issue.

> Obesity is widespread, associated with several physical and psychosocial comorbidities, and is difficult to treat. Prevention of obesity across the lifespan is critical to improving the health of individuals and society. Screening and prevention efforts in primary care are an important step in addressing the obesity epidemic. Each period of human development is associated with unique risks, challenges, and opportunities for prevention and intervention. Screening tools for overweight/obesity, although imperfect, are quick and easy to administer. Screening should be conducted at every primary care visit and tracked longitudinally. Screening tools and cutoffs for overweight and obesity vary by age group.

With the growing obesity epidemic, it is difficult for individual primary care providers to devote the time and effort necessary to achieve meaningful weight loss for significant numbers of patients. A variety of health care professionals provide value and evidence-based care that is effective in treating obesity and other preventable diseases. Multidisciplinary collaboration between primary care physicians and other trained health professionals within patient-centered medical homes offers an effective approach to sustainable behavioral treatment options for individuals who are obese or overweight.

Medications for obesity management can be divided into 4 groups: antidepressants (naltrexone/bupropion), stimulants (phentermine, phendimetrazine, diethylpropion, phentermine/topiramate), fat blockers (orlistat), and diabetes medications (liraglutide). Each group has specific therapeutic effects, adverse effects, and costs. Two medications are indicated for long-term use in obesity: lorcaserin and orlistat. Other available medications are for short-term use. High cost makes many of these medications inaccessible for underserved and poor patients. Because of misuse potential, many obesity medications are also classified as controlled substances. There are no medications currently approved for use in pregnant or lactating women.

This article provides the reader with steps needed to accurately assess patient nutrition behaviors that contribute to weight gain, inability to lose weight, or inability to sustain weight loss. Evidence-based approaches in nutrition therapy that can create the daily energy deficit needed to produce 1/2 to 2 pounds of weight loss per week, and the strategies to create the energy deficit, are presented. To optimize health, long-term weight loss maintenance is needed. The benefits of using a multidisciplinary team approach in treating obesity are highlighted.

Parallel to rising obesity rates is an increase in costs associated with excess weight. Estimates of future direct (medical) and indirect (nonmedical) costs related to obesity suggest rising expenditures that will impose a significant economic burden to individuals and society as a whole. This article reviews research on direct and indirect medical costs and future economic trends associated with obesity and associated comorbidities. Cost disparities associated with subsets of the population experiencing higher than average rates of obesity are explored. Finally, potential solutions with the highest estimated impact are offered, and future directions are proposed.

Impacts of Physical Activity on the Obese   97

Meshia Q. Waleh

Approximately two-thirds of the US population is overweight or obese. Physical activity is recommended for preventing obesity, aiding in weight loss, and decreasing rates of chronic diseases. This article reviews current statistics for obesity, physical activity, and physician counseling patterns. Principles of exercise physiology relating to cardiopulmonary fitness and chronic disease are also reviewed, and methods for increasing physical activity in adults and children are suggested.

Obesity in Special Populations: Pregnancy   109

Danielle Symons Downs

Perinatal overweight and obesity is a major public health and clinical care issue that requires deliberate and immediate attention. Preconception and prenatal assessment and counseling should address the risks associated with obesity, recommendations for weight gain, proper nutrition and dietary intake, and physical activity. Nutrition and exercise guidance should be offered to all perinatal overweight and obese women with an emphasis on effective strategies to overcome barriers. All women should be encouraged to adopt a healthy lifestyle and achieve a healthy weight before becoming pregnant.

Obesity Statistics   121

Kristy Breuhl Smith and Michael Seth Smith

Obesity is a chronic disease that is strongly associated with an increase in mortality and morbidity including certain types of cancer, cardiovascular disease, disability, diabetes mellitus, hypertension, osteoarthritis, and stroke. In adults, overweight is defined as a body mass index (BMI) of 25 kg/m^2 to 29 kg/m^2 and obesity as a BMI of greater than 30 kg/m^2. If current trends continue, it is estimated that, by the year 2030, 38% of the world's adult population will be overweight and another 20% obese. Significant global health strategies must reduce the morbidity and mortality associated with the obesity epidemic.

Obesity in Older Adults   137

Virginia B. Kalish

The percentage of older obese adults is on the rise. Many clinicians underestimate the health consequences of obesity in the elderly, citing scarce evidence and concerns that weight loss might be detrimental to the health of older adults. Although overweight and obese elders are not at the same risk for morbidity and mortality as younger individuals, quality of life and function are adversely impacted. Weight loss plans in the elderly should include aerobic activities as well as balance and resistance activities to maintain optimal physical function.

PRIMARY CARE:
CLINICS IN OFFICE PRACTICE

THE CLINICS ARE AVAILABLE ONLINE!
Access your subscription at:
www.theclinics.com

PRIMARY CARE:
CLINICS IN OFFICE PRACTICE

Foreword
Just Eat Less and Exercise More?

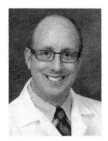

Joel J. Heidelbaugh, MD, FAAFP, FACG
Consulting Editor

It is with great excitement that I present this issue of *Primary Care: Clinics in Office Practice* dedicated to the topic of obesity management, which remains a prevailing challenge in our daily practices, and a perennial national health care crisis. While national societies have developed guidelines, and various interest groups have created many useful provisions for strategic education and intervention, the pediatric and adult obesity rates in the United States remain alarming. We, the ever-busy health care practitioners, are perfectly skilled in sheepishly telling our patients to *"just eat less and exercise more,"* which rarely cuts the mustard (sorry, I couldn't resist...). We also still fall well short of providing preprofessional (Liaison Committee on Medical Education nutrition education requirement is less than 5 hours over 4 years) and resident education on HOW to motivate and educate our obese patients toward reasonable weight loss goals and HOW to empower them to be successful.

The concept and causation of obesity absolutely fascinate me. Thinking back to high school in the 1980s, I can think of only a few kids in my school who were really obese, and that would likely pale in comparison to obesity standards today. We all imbibed soda, ate chips and cookies, and watched MTV, video games, and other garbage, and somehow didn't become obese to the extent that kids are today. So what has changed? Are kids today just eating more bad calories and getting less exercise? Are there genetic switches that have been activated to modify hormone regulation through environmental factors that we haven't identified and developed drugs to combat?

A recent well-child examination for a 12-year-old, 5-foot, 4-inch, 266-pound (BMI 45.7) asthmatic boy presented this difficult discussion with his mother: *"Dr. H, you've gotta tell my son to stop eating so much. He won't listen to me. I found cookies under his bed and empty soda bottles on the floor. He watches too much television and constantly plays video games on his cell phone. It's impossible to get him to do his homework. He complains when I give him vegetables. Every day after school he wants me to take him to McDonald's because he's hungry".*

Prim Care Clin Office Pract 43 (2016) xiii–xiv
http://dx.doi.org/10.1016/j.pop.2015.10.006   **primarycare.theclinics.com**
0095-4543/16/$ – see front matter © 2016 Published by Elsevier Inc.

So, what would you do? How effective do you think you can be in motivating and educating this child to make changes? How would you teach his mother to take control by creating dietary and activity limitations for her son? How would you feel about having a child with pediatric obesity on your patient panel, for which you are held accountable for outcomes under the provisions of population management?

This issue of *Primary Care: Clinics in Office Practice* begins with a summary of harrowing statistics on obesity, much of which we already know, but which are presented in a novel fashion that allow us to better understand the data on who are most susceptible and afflicted by obesity and comorbid factors. The next article details the economic burden of obesity, again which we can likely estimate, but continually underestimate and often take for granted that it will just multiply. We all play a role in prevention on the "micro," or patient-to-patient level, yet will now have enhanced knowledge and skills to become better advocates for the "macro" level change in our communities. The article on national health care policy on obesity management is outstanding, with a review of current strategies for legislation and changes in food manufacturing and preparation.

The article that highlights the model of the patient-centered medical home provides an exemplary construct for a multidisciplinary approach toward obesity management. This includes utilizing our resources of health educators and coaches, dietitians, and exercise physiologists, coupled with harnessing our own potential for obesity education and management. These principles play key roles across all populations, from children and adolescents to adults, including pregnant women. The promise of pharmacologic management is reviewed, as novel therapies are presented with reference to their basis in pathophysiology and endocrinology. Last, a review of surgical therapies for obesity is provided, highlighting vast successes in weight loss management over the last few decades, with rapid advancements in surgical techniques and impressive decreases in morbidity and mortality rates.

I would like to thank Dr Mark Stephens and his authors for creating a wonderful compendium of articles on the important topic of obesity management. As usual, I Googled many of the authors of the articles within this issue to learn about their expertise. Impressively, all are highly visible experts in the fields of clinical medicine and surgery with a focus on nutrition and epidemiology centered on teaching, creating written and video educational tools, and promoting public health initiatives to combat obesity. This issue provides a substantial amount of useful information for the practicing clinician, researcher, and medical educator. What I gained most from this issue is that we can collectively become greater motivating factors in our patient's lives and partner with them to lose weight and improve their health outcomes. I'll never look at another tortilla chip or video game the same way again....

Joel J. Heidelbaugh, MD, FAAFP, FACG
Departments of Family Medicine and Urology
University of Michigan Medical School
Ann Arbor, MI 48109, USA

Ypsilanti Health Center
200 Arnet Suite 200
Ypsilanti, MI 48198, USA

E-mail address:
jheidel@umich.edu

Preface

Obesity: A Plague Upon Our Houses

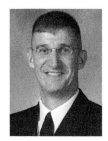

Mark B. Stephens, MD, MS, FAAFP, CAPT, MC, USN
Editor

One in three American adults is obese. The direct and indirect costs associated with obesity and relevant comorbidities are staggering. While multiple primary, secondary, and tertiary approaches have been developed to combat the issue of overweight and obesity, the "secret sauce" has yet to be discovered. Obesity is a multifactorial disease with complex genetic, environmental, and social factors. The modern American environment is increasingly obesogenic. Stigmatization and bias contribute to inequalities in health care outcomes. It is with this context in mind that the present issue was designed to help practicing clinicians understand some of the complex, interrelated issues impacting the treatment of obesity (from individual patient through national policy) across the lifespan. The first two articles provide background data about general obesity statistics and the economic impact of America's expanding waistline. The third article is dedicated to pediatric obesity. The following articles review screening, behavioral modification, nutritional therapy, and physical activity as fundamental elements of any obesity-related program. Advances in the pharmacologic and surgical approaches to obesity are reviewed in the next two articles, followed by two articles that use the context of the patient-centered medical home and the changing health care landscape to offer thoughtful insights regarding policymaking and a systematic national approach to the obesity epidemic. The issue closes with a review of obesity in pregnancy and the aging population.

Mark B. Stephens, MD, MS, FAAFP, CAPT, MC, USN
Department of Family Medicine
Uniformed Services University
4301 Jones Bridge Road
Bethesda, MD 20814, USA

E-mail address:
mark.stephens@usuhs.edu

Prim Care Clin Office Pract 43 (2016) xv
http://dx.doi.org/10.1016/j.pop.2015.10.005
0095-4543/16/$ – see front matter © 2016 Published by Elsevier Inc.

primarycare.theclinics.com

The Future of Pediatric Obesity

Jeff Hutchinson, MD[a],*, Jill Emerick, MD[b], Harshita Saxena, MD[b]

KEYWORDS

- Obesity • Social media • Nutrition • Peer influence • Physical activity
- Wearable technology • Motivational interviewing

KEY POINTS

- Obesity has increased over the last 30 years across the nation and disproportionately in the Latino and black cultures.
- Food marketing targets vulnerable children and adolescents but can be countered by education.
- Emerging technology may benefit children and adolescents in attaining healthier lifestyles.
- The pediatric multidisciplinary approach is unique and requires a family-centered approach.
- Treatment options are a challenging evolution in the pediatric population with behavioral modification as the foundation of success.

INTRODUCTION AND OVERVIEW OF CHILDHOOD OBESITY
Providers Struggle with Obesity Treatment

The medical community has been aware of the pediatric obesity epidemic for over a decade and yet providers self-report a low degree of confidence in their ability to successfully treat childhood obesity. Only 30% of general pediatricians feel they are good to excellent at providing obesity counseling and only 10% feel that their counseling is effective.[1] In 2007, expert committee recommendations (ECRs) regarding the prevention, assessment, and treatment of child and adolescent overweight and obesity were published.[2] Despite these ECRs, counseling given during well visits at the primary care practice level has not significantly changed. The frequency of lifestyle counseling for patients has not changed, and socioeconomically disadvantaged children diagnosed with obesity have received counseling less frequently since the ECRs were published.[3] These findings highlight some of the difficulties providers face in trying to incorporate obesity prevention and healthy lifestyle counseling into daily practice.

[a] Department of Pediatrics, Uniformed Services University, 4301 Jones Bridge Road, Bethesda, MD 20814, USA; [b] Department of Pediatrics, Walter Reed National Military Medical Center, 8901 Rockville Pike, Bethesda, MD 20889, USA
* Corresponding author.
E-mail address: JHutchinson@usuhs.edu

Prim Care Clin Office Pract 43 (2016) 1–17
http://dx.doi.org/10.1016/j.pop.2015.08.007   primarycare.theclinics.com
0095-4543/16/$ – see front matter Published by Elsevier Inc.

Prevalence of Childhood Obesity

Childhood obesity is defined as a body mass index (BMI) at or above sex- and age-specific 95th percentile norms from the 2000 Centers for Disease Control and Prevention (CDC) Growth Charts. The prevalence of childhood obesity has increased since 1993 but has not changed significantly for most groups since 2003 to 2004, remaining at current levels of around 17%.[4] There have even been nationwide improvements in some areas. Improvements include a reduction in obesity rates in 2 to 5 year olds from 13.9% in 2003 to 2004 to 8.4% in 2011 to 2012. This success is likely attributable to multiple efforts.[5]

Trends Among Age Groups

Fig. 1 shows obesity trends by age group. A greater percentage of black and Latino children are classified as obese.

Cultural Considerations with Weight

Obesity is influenced by multiple and complex factors. In the simplest terms, weight gain and weight loss are determined by overall energy balance as determined by caloric intake and caloric expenditure. For children and their families, language, culture, and environment interact to influence intake and expenditure and motivation to change behaviors. The disproportionate increase in obesity among certain ethnic groups (often despite income) challenges providers to consider their personal biases, expectations, and assumptions when planning patient- and family-specific interventions.[6]

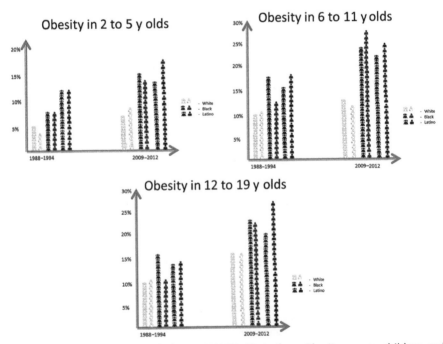

Fig. 1. Childhood obesity trends from NHANES. (*Data from* Obesity among children and adolescents aged 2–19 years, by selected characteristics: United States, selected years 1988–1994 through 2009–2012. National Center for Health Statistics. Centers for Disease Control and Prevention. Available at: http://www.cdc.gov/nchs/data/hus/2014/065.pdf. Accessed June 28, 2015.)

The specific words and language used to discuss weight matters. "Overweight," "heavy," "fat," and "obese" may elicit different emotional responses. Words like "husky" may have a judgmental tone, while words such as "healthy" or "heavy set" in the black culture may normalize being overweight or obese. Language can remove or perpetuate the stigma of obesity and influence medical care. Removing fear and stigma with purposeful communication can improve a patient's desire to access health care and contribute to a plan for healthier behavior. **Table 1** illustrates strategies for cultural awareness in the context of weight management.

Table 1 Cultural awareness strategies	
Avoid stereotypes and assumptions	"What do you think of your child's/your weight?"
Acknowledge past experiences and efforts	"What have you been told? What have you tried? What made a difference?"
Focus on the behavior not the weight	Ask yourself: "Am I treating the patient or the condition?" "Can traditional food become healthier?" Avoid a weight discussion with every encounter. A visit for a cold should not become focused on weight
Have a supportive environment	Be aware of media and furniture that make obese patients feel unwanted Have appropriately sized equipment (blood pressure cuffs and larger gowns) readily available Obtain vitals such as weight and height metrics in a private setting
Give concrete advice preferably confirming the patient/parent's plan	Ask: "What do you want to try now until the next time I see you again?"

Special Considerations in Adolescents

Growing children and adolescents often turn to peers for information and advice as they explore their independence and strive to form their identities. Young patients are subject to both positive and negative messages from peers and media. Print media, in particular, perpetuate unrealistic notions of the perfect body through image manipulation, and nonrepresentative models that add additional pressures to highly susceptible youth.[7] After successful weight loss, adolescents are at high risk of disordered eating and can battle with poor self-esteem and body image that can make treatment more challenging. Physicians cognizant of these pressures can learn to provide empathetic and meaningful care to their patients by considering the whole patient and recognizing comorbid conditions such as depression, low resilience, substance use, and bullying. Confidential one-on-one care often facilitates children and adolescents in their move toward changing behaviors in a healthy way, and adolescents especially benefit from independent time with a provider every visit.[8] In the end, parents remain the source with the most direct influence on adolescent behavior.

A CLINICAL APPROACH TO CHILDHOOD OBESITY

Despite wanting to improve their obesity intervention skills, most practitioners lack confidence and do not bring up obesity during a patient encounter.[9] The following section offers a practical approach to pediatric obesity (**Fig. 2**).

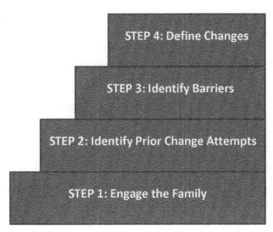

Fig. 2. Steps to approach obesity.

Step 1: Engage the Family

Choosing the appropriate setting to discuss weight management is important. Rapport is essential to engage in the topic if obesity is not the intended purpose of the visit. Discussing weight unexpectedly may alienate patients and make them less likely to seek care.[10] Well-child visits and routine physical examinations (eg, sports physicals) are good opportunities to discuss this topic. Directly asking if there are any concerns about the child's weight is a good place to start.

Step 2: Identify Previous Attempts to Change

It is important to determine if the family has previously made any attempts to change weight or adopt a healthier lifestyle. Further probing questions might include the following:

- How did their past interventions work?
- Were they able to maintain the changes?
- How did they feel while working on their stated behavior?
- If they were unable to maintain change, what got in their way?
- If they have not tried anything in the past, what would it take to alter unhealthy behaviors?

Using simple techniques of motivational interviewing (MI), the answers to these questions provide a sense of the patient's past successes and challenges on their journey to healthier habits and also allows for shared insight into potential strategies for behavioral change.

Step 3: Identify Barriers to Behavior Change

Table 2 lists several common barriers to change. Assessing the patient's readiness to change is important when identifying potential barriers. Overcoming barriers depends on how ready the patient and family are to make a change (see **Table 2**). Families that have attempted change likely have insight into past barriers and may be more receptive to discussing new strategies to overcome these obstacles. Barriers identified by the patient are as important as barriers identified by the family.[11,12]

Table 2 Barriers to weight loss	
Provider Listed Barriers	**Patient Listed Barriers**
Lack of patient or parent motivation to change	No perceived need for treatment
Lack of parental concern	No perceived need for further changes
Too much fast food	Treatment perceived as not efficacious
Too much screen time	Participation barriers
Not enough exercise	Situational factors
Provider low confidence in creating change	Fear of stigma

Adapted from Spivack J, Swietlik M, Alessandrini E, et al. Primary care providers' knowledge, practices, and perceived barriers to the treatment and prevention of childhood obesity. Obesity (Silver Spring) 2010;18(7):1341–7; and Perez A, Holt N, Gokiert R, et al. Why don't families initiate treatment? A qualitative multicenter study investigating parents' reasons for declining paediatric weight management. Paediatr Child Health 2015;20(4):179–84.

Step 4: Help the Patient and Family Define Important Changes

Patients and families should choose a priority and strategize how to effectively incorporate agreed on changes or goals into their daily life. Goals should be *SMART* (Specific, Measurable, Attainable, Realistic, and Timely).[13] For example, an SMART goal is "I will walk for 60 minutes, 5 days a week for the next month," *not* "I need to exercise more." Review barriers to achieving this goal and proactively plan ways to overcome them.

History and Physical Examination

As part of a comprehensive medical history, it is important to identify the presence of or risk for comorbid conditions. A 3-generation pedigree family history will identify potential underlying genetic risk for many comorbid illnesses (diabetes, cardiovascular disease) and provide insight into heritable somatotype. Inquire about prior medication use (**Table 3**).

Table 3 Medications that affect weight	
Weight Change Profile of Medications Commonly Used in Pediatrics	
Weight Gain Promoting Medication	
Insulin	Antipsychotics
Tricyclic antidepressants	Haloperidol
Amitriptyline	Loxapine
Doxepin	Clozapine
Imipramine	Chlorpromazine
Nortriptyline	Fluphenazine
Trimipramine	Resperidone
Mirtazapine	Olanzapine
Selective serotonin reuptake inhibitors	Quetiapine
Sertraline	Antiseizure
Paroxetine	Valproic acid
Fluvoxamine	Carbamazepine
Lithium	Gabapentin
β-Adrenergic blockers	Oral corticosteroids
Estrogens and Progestins	Inhaled corticosteroids (high dose)
	Antihistamines

(continued on next page)

Table 3
(continued)
Weight Change Profile of Medications Commonly Used in Pediatrics
Weight loss promoting

Stimulants	Metformin
Methylphenidate	Topiramate
Amphetamine	
Dextroamphetamine	
Dexmethylphenidate	
Lisdexamfetamine	

The physical examination includes standard measures of height and weight and vital signs with every focused or general physical examination with additional awareness of findings found in **Table 5**. In addition, BMI is calculated, and waist circumference may be useful.

Body mass index vs waist circumference

BMI is calculated by dividing a person's weight in kilograms by the square of their height in meters.

BMI percentile calculator for child and teen (English version): http://nccd.cdc.gov/dnpabmi/Calculator.aspx.

Waist circumference measurement

To correctly measure waist circumference (**Fig. 3**, **Table 4**):

- Stand and place a tape measure around the waist, just above the hipbones
- Make sure tape is horizontal around the waist
- Keep the tape snug around the waist, but not compressing the skin
- Measure the waist just after the patient breathes out
- Compare to anthropomorphic standards[14]

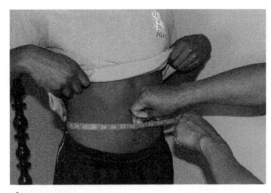

Fig. 3. Waist circumference measurement.

BMI and waist circumference can indicate a high amount of body fat. Both can be used as screening tools to determine the need for further evaluation or intervention.

As outlined by the childhood obesity algorithm (**Fig. 4**), laboratory screening is based on BMI and age. For children with a healthy weight (BMI 5%–84%), assess medical and behavioral risks for developing an unhealthy weight, provide prevention counseling, and reassess weight velocity at subsequent visits. Children with BMI

Table 4
90th percentile waist circumference in centimeters by age and sex

Age	6	7	8	9	10	11	12	13	14	15	16	17	18
Boys	69.6	71.3	78.1	85	85.6	90.4	93.7	96.7	101.3	99.9	106.1	108	105.9
Girls	64.3	72.9	78.7	83	84.1	93.6	95.1	96.8	94.4	101.4	102.2	99.5	107.1

From Fryar CD, Gu Q, Ogden CL. Anthropometric reference data for children and adults: United States, 2007–2010. National Center for Health Statistics. Vital Health Stat 2012;11(252):1–48. Available at: http://www.cdc.gov/nchs/data/series/sr_11/sr11_252.pdf.

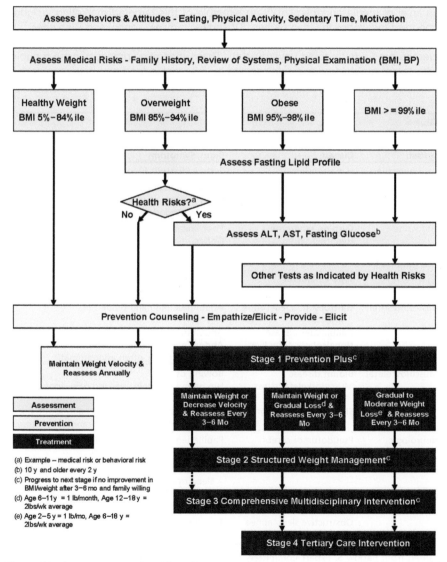

Fig. 4. Obesity assessment algorithm. (*Courtesy of* National Institute for Children's Health Quality (NICHQ), Boston, MA; with permission.)

greater than the 85th percentile should be screened for comorbid conditions such as hyperlipidemia, type 2 diabetes, and nonalcoholic fatty liver disease because these may develop without other signs or symptoms.

Some obesity-related diagnoses present more rapidly, and clues are evident on history and physical examination. **Table 5** outlines common related diagnoses by system.

More About Barriers: Media Influence and Pediatric Obesity

Media and marketing strategies are significant challenges in obesity prevention and treatment. Brain maturation continues into the teen and young adult years. Twelve to 14 year olds are especially impacted as they increase independence and have a high level of media engagement.[15] An example of this targeted marketing includes embedded messages in video games, TV shows, movies, songs, and Web sites.[16]

The food and beverage industry spends up to $2 billion annually on food and beverage products targeted toward youth. These marketing practices pose a public health threat for children and adolescents by influencing food and beverage preferences, purchases, and consumption.[17]

Table 5		
Obesity related diagnoses		
System	**Disease**	**Signs/Symptoms**
Cardiovascular	Hypertension	Systolic/diastolic blood pressure >95% for age and height
Genetic	Prader-Willi syndrome	Short stature, primary amenorrhea, undescended testes, small hands and feet
Endocrine	Cushing syndrome	Poor linear growth, violaceous striae
	Hypothyroidism	Goiter
	Polycystic ovary syndrome	Excessive acne, hirsutism, irregular menses, primary amenorrhea
	Type 2 diabetes	Acanthosis nigricans, polyuria, polydypsia, unexpected weight loss
Gastrointestinal	Gastroesophageal reflux disease	Abdominal pain and tenderness
	Gallbladder disease	Abdominal pain and tenderness
	Nonalcoholic fatty liver disease	Abdominal pain and tenderness, hepatomegaly, often asymptomatic
Musculoskeletal	Blount disease	Bowing of tibia
	Musculoskeletal stress from weight	Hip pain, knee pain, walking pain, foot pain
	Slipped capital femoral epiphysis	Hip pain, knee pain, walking pain, foot pain, abnormal gait, limited hip range of motion
Neurologic	Pseudotumor cerebri	Papilledema, cranial nerve VI paralysis, severe recurrent headaches
Psychological	Depression	Anxiety, school avoidance, social isolation, sleepiness and wakefulness
Pulmonary	Asthma	Wheezing, shortness of breath, exercise intolerance
	Obstructive sleep apnea	Tonsillar hypertrophy, snoring, apnea, daytime sleepiness, nocturnal enuresis

Adapted from Barlow S, Expert Committee. Expert committee recommendations regarding the prevention, assessment, and treatment of child and adolescent overweight and obesity: summary report. Pediatrics 2007;120;S164.

Most food and beverages advertised on children's Web sites are unhealthy. More than 80% of advertised products are excessively high in fat, sugar, and/or sodium.[18] About 1.2 million children play industry-sponsored games (advergames) every month. Food marketing (often unhealthy products, such as candies, chips, and sugar-sweetened beverages) is omnipresent at school, athletic events, and music events.[19,20] Children and adolescents are also exposed to professional athlete and celebrity product endorsements.[21]

The World Health Organization recommends policies to limit young people's exposure to food advertisements.[22] The impact of advertising healthier options is difficult to assess because companies use different criteria and inconsistent nutritional standards.[23] Industry self-regulation has not led to significant improvements in the nutritional quality of foods marketed to youth. Companies continue to aggressively market to older (yet still vulnerable) children and adolescents.[15,24]

Technology as a Tool Against Obesity: Social Marketing

Social marketing strategies can counter aggressive food and beverage industry tactics by applying common commercial marketing principles for the benefit of the intended audience.[25] Examples are presented in **Table 6**. Parental and community role modeling and positive images of healthy behaviors can be useful if children are the focus.[26] The CDC's "VERB" Campaign is an example of an effective tool that branded children's play as socially desirable and helped increase preadolescent physical activity.[27,28] Celebrity endorsements such as the "Got Milk" campaign can also help rebrand healthy food products and appeal to youth.

Technology as a Tool Against Obesity: Wearable Technology and Applications

Wearable fitness trackers and device applications offer additional strategies to health care providers to assist pediatric patients struggling with weight issues. Wearable devices record periods of activity and inactivity throughout the day. They provide passive

Table 6
Campaigns for obesity prevention

Social Marketing for Childhood Obesity Prevention		
Got Milk Campaign and now the Milk Life campaign	California Milk Processor Board 1993	http://adage.com/article/news/milk-dropped-national-milk-industry-tactics/291819/
CDC Verb It's What You Do campaign 2002–2006	Effective at increasing preadolescent physical activity (Berkowitz)	http://www.cdc.gov/youthcampaign/
5-4-3-2-1-Go!	Consortium to lower obesity in Chicago Children: targets adults, especially parents because parents are "agents of change" in childhood obesity	http://www.clocc.net/
Let's Move campaign	Initiated by Michelle Obama	http://www.letsmove.gov/
9-5-2-1-0 Let's Go BFF! 5-2-1-0 campaign	Safe & Healthy Children's Coalition	http://www.safehealthychildren.org/95210-lets-go-2/ http://www.letsgo.org/

Adapted from Evans WD, Christoffel KK, Mecheles JW, et al. Social marketing as a childhood obesity prevention strategy. Obesity 2010;18(1):s23–6.

messages of encouragement to patients striving to meet specific activity goals. Studies show that children who use fitness tracking technology are more likely to engage in moderate to vigorous physical activity.[29]

Smartphone applications sending ongoing reminders to users are available to achieve fitness goals. Such applications can promote higher participant activity levels.[30,31] Individuals using fitness applications have been shown to eat less fast food, exercise more, reduce screen time, and have a greater awareness of knowledge of daily vegetable consumption.[32]

There is also a market for video games to encourage physical activity. Games estimating physical activity may serve as a useful tool to inform parents and children about estimated activity levels, reduce advergame use, and also motivate children to achieve set activity goals.[32]

Technology as a Tool Against obesity: The Use of Social Media

Adolescents are receptive to receiving online information, such as recipes, weight loss tips, and health-related quizzes. They are also open to live chats with providers. Two-thirds of adolescents aged 13 to 17 use Facebook, and there has been discussion about a weight management group for adolescents on this social media platform.[33] Privacy issues remain a concern, and most adolescents would prefer a separate parent-focused page to maintain confidentiality.

Text messaging can be used to encourage healthier lifestyles to achieve weight goals. Tailored short-message service (SMS) scripts effectively promote positive health-related behavioral changes in adults. SMS holds promise for encouraging healthy behaviors in older children and adolescents as well. Social media outreach and text messaging are helpful adjuncts to existing multidisciplinary obesity treatment interventions.[34]

Treatment Stages

ECRs regarding the prevention, assessment, and treatment of child and adolescent overweight and obesity recommended a stratified treatment approach.

Stage 1 (Prevention Plus) defines the interaction between patient, family, and care team with special emphasis on healthy eating and activity habits.[2] The 5-2-1-0 Let's Go program is a sample of a nationally recognized childhood obesity prevention program initiated in Maine and a few neighboring states (http://letsgo.org). The prescription for healthy living is based on the 5-2-1-0 mnemonic (5 servings of fruits and vegetables; no more than 2 hours of screen time a day; at least 1 hour of physical activity daily; and zero sugar-sweetened beverages). This prescription serves as one template for a Prevention Plus interaction. The 5-2-1-0 program has been expanded by The Fit Kids 360 curriculum to the 8-7-6-5-4-3-2-1-0 prescription (**Table 7**).[35]

MI techniques help during the early phases of obesity treatment. The basics of MI include exploring pros and cons of proposed behaviors by using a reflective listening approach to engage resistance or ambivalence by asking further questions rather than proposing rote solutions. MI emphasizes shared decision-making and agenda setting. MI is a learned skill with basic principles designed to identify and address successes and barriers to changing behavior.[36] MI helps families prioritize goals and determine follow-up needs. The goal is to stimulate behavior change by assessing motivating factors for the patient rather than encouraging behavior change based simply on information passed from provider to patient.[37]

Change Talk (https://www.youtube.com/watch?v=HFUvEZI9mjE), an initiative of the American Academy of Pediatrics, is an online mobile app designed to provide

Table 7
Prescription for healthy living

8-7-6-5-4-3-2-1-0 Prescription for Healthy Living	
8	8–11 h of sleep each night
7	7 breakfasts every week
6	6 home-cooked meals around the table every week
5	5 servings of fruit and vegetables every day
4	4 positive self-messages every day
3	3 servings of low fat dairy daily
2	2 h or less of screen time daily
1	1 hour or more of physical activity daily
0	0 sugar-sweetened beverages per day

From Tucker J, Eisenmann J, Howard K, et al. FitKids360: design, conduct, and outcomes of a stage 2 pediatric obesity program. J Obes 2014;2014:37404.

virtual assistance to providers to hone motivational interviewing skills. If patients fail to progress toward a healthier BMI after 3 to 6 months of a Prevention Plus intervention, moving to a stage 2: intervention (Structured Weight Management program) is recommended.

Stage 2 (Structured Weight Management) programs include the assistance of a dietician or nutritionist to assist with structured meal planning. Enhanced emphasis of reduced screen time to (less than 1 hour per day) and an increase in planned or supervised physical activity to at least 60 minutes a day are recommended. Exercise specialists can help guide and plan physical activities, and behavioral health professionals can help parents and patients in their approach to developing healthy lifestyle by promoting cognitive skills and resolving family conflicts and other relationship issues. Log books can provide helpful information about diet, physical activity, and ongoing barriers to change. Monthly office visits help monitor behavior change and provide ongoing positive reinforcement.[2] A significant decrease in BMI and BMI z-scores have been demonstrated with a 7-week stage 2 program.[38]

Stage 3 (Comprehensive Multidisciplinary Intervention) intensifies treatment even further, optimally in a group setting with providers from multiple disciplines. Team members may include a behavioral counselor, registered dietitian, exercise specialist, and primary care provider. Stage 3 occurs outside of the primary care office and typically involves 8 to 12 weekly meetings to help initiate behavior change. Subsequent monthly visits help to maintain positive changes.[2] Early intervention may lead to more successful obesity treatment, particularly in children under the age of 5.[36]

A comprehensive "Healthy Habits Clinic" provides multiple benefits to the patient and family, including peer support and the participation of multiple family members to encourage familial change rather than individual change. Obesity runs in families, and parental obesity is a known risk factor for childhood obesity.[30] Approaching obesity treatment as a family increases the likelihood for successful behavior change and provides the unique opportunity for simultaneous treatment of obese parents and children. Family-based therapy allows for a significant cost savings and weight loss in parents, and percent BMI reduction in children is significantly greater in family-based therapy.[39] Comprehensive obesity clinics allow for medical treatment, nutrition education, exercise, and behavioral health within the context of a single visit.

Table 8
Weight loss medications: pharmacologic agents approved for obesity treatment

Drug	US Food and Drug Administration–approved Obesity Drugs			
	Approved Age	Mechanism of Action	Placebo-Subtracted Weight Loss in Phase 3 Trials	Common Adverse Effects	Contraindications
Orlistat (Xenical) • 120 mg orally 3 times daily • Immediately before, during, or after meals	12	Intestinal lipase inhibitor	3.0%	• Oily stools • Malabsorption of fat-soluble vitamins • Multivitamins recommended	• Malabsorption syndrome • Cholestasis • Pregnancy/breast-feeding
Lorcaserin (Belviq) • 10 mg twice daily	Adult One study in 12–17 y olds; results not yet available[a]	5-hydroxytryptamine (serotonin) receptor 2C agonist	3.0%–3.6%	Headache, nausea, dry mouth, dizziness, fatigue, constipation	• Selective serotonin reuptake/Serotonin and norepinephrine reuptake inhibitor and related drugs • Coexisting congestive cardiac failure • Valvulopathy • Pregnancy
Phentiramine/topiramate (Qsymia) • Starting dose 3.75 mg/23 mg daily • Standard maintenance dose 7.5 mg/46 mg daily • Highest dose 15 mg/92 mg daily	Adult One retrospective chart review of adolescents up to age 18 showed 4%–6% reduction of BMI over 6 mo with topiramate and lifestyle changes[45,46]	Norepinephrine + dopamine release/ GABA modulation	6.6% at standard dose 8.6%–9.3% at highest dose	Paresthesia, dizziness, altered taste, insomnia, constipation, dry mouth	• Pregnancy • Recent or unstable cardiovascular disease • Glaucoma • Hyperthyroidism • Monoamine oxidase inhibitors or sympathomimetic amines

[a] Arena Pharmaceuticals. Single dose study to determine the safety, tolerability, and pharmacokinetic properties of Lorcaserin hydrochloride (Belviq) in obese adolescents from 12 to 17 years of age [identifier: NCT02022956]. Available at: http://clinicaltrials.gov/show/NVT2022956. Accessed June 24, 2015.

Adapted from Jones BJ, Bloom SR. The new era of drug therapy for obesity: the evidence and the expectations. Drugs 2015;75(9):940; with permission.

Stage 4 (Tertiary Care Intervention) should be considered for severely obese youth who have attempted weight control in the comprehensive multidisciplinary intervention stage, have the maturity to understand possible risks, and are willing to maintain physical activity, a healthy diet, and appropriate behavioral monitoring. Stage 4 interventions include the consideration of the use of a very low calorie diet only in children finished growing, medications, and weight control surgery.[2]

Medications for Childhood Obesity

There is one medication approved for use in patients age 12 and over. Orlistat is an intestinal lipase inhibitor that showed a sustained weight loss of 3% over placebo when given at the standard dose of 120 mg 3 times daily.[40] Reduced progression to diabetes and improved glycemic control in known diabetics have also been shown in patients taking orlistat for weight loss.[41,42] Alli is the over-the-counter formulation of orlistat and is packaged to be dosed as 60 mg with meals 3 times a day. Orlistat works by blocking intestinal fat absorption. As a result, common gastrointestinal side effects include oily stools, fecal urgency, fecal leakage, and spotting.[43] Side effects are worse if patients consume higher levels of fat, but generally improve after the first several weeks of treatment. It is hypothesized that some of the effectiveness of orlistat stems from dietary changes made to avoid side effects as opposed to solely reduced caloric absorption.[44]

With the growing obesity epidemic, there is increasing pressure for pharmaceutical companies to develop more products. Since 2012, 4 new weight loss medications have been approved for use in adults (**Table 8**). Three of these newly approved agents

Table 9	
Bariatric surgery considerations	
Consider if:	
BMI $\geq$35 kg/m^2	BMI >40 kg/m^2
PLUS at least one serious comorbidity:	PLUS other comorbidities:
• Type 2 diabetes mellitus	• Insulin resistance or glucose intolerance
• Moderate to severe obstructive sleep apnea	• Mild obstructive sleep apnea
• Pseudotumor cerebri	• Hypertension
• Severe steatohepatitis	• Hyperlipidemia
	• Impaired weight-related quality of life
Recommended for all adolescent surgical candidates	
Sexual maturity rating Tanner IV or V or bone age greater than or equal to 13 in girls and greater than or equal to 15 in boys	
Able to provide informed assent	
At least 6 mo of attempted weight loss without success	
Able to understand and comply with lifestyle changes required postoperatively (dietary, physical activity, supplementation, medical follow-up)	
Contraindications to bariatric surgery	
The adolescent:	
• Has a medically correctable cause of obesity	
• Has a substance abuse problem in the preceding year	
• Is unable to understand or unwilling to commit to the surgery as well as presurgical and postsurgical regimen	
• Is pregnant, plans to become pregnant soon after the surgery, or is lactating as a result of recent pregnancy	

Adapted from Inge TH, Krebs KF, Barcia VF, et al. Bariatric surgery for severely overweight adolescents: concerns and recommendations. Pediatrics 2004;11:217–23.

have been studied in adolescents: lorcaserin, topiramate (alone, not in combination with phentiramine), and liraglutide. The results of the topiramate and liraglutide studies show weight loss in adolescents similar to that seen in adult patients.[45,46] All of the approved medications are adjuncts to ongoing healthy lifestyle and behavioral changes.

Surgical Treatment of Obesity in Adolescents

Bariatric surgery is a limited therapy available for carefully selected adolescents (**Table 9**).[47]

SUMMARY

Overcoming childhood and adolescent obesity requires family engagement, a multidisciplinary approach, addressing cultural norms, and using technology as a tool. Future treatment strategies to combat obesity will include efforts beyond the health care provider's office, including media, appropriate legislation, and the broad involvement of the educational system. Despite the high likelihood that future physicians will have a wider variety of medications and safer surgical procedures in their obesity treatment tool kit, behavior modification and healthy lifestyle changes remain the key components to successful pediatric obesity prevention and treatment.

REFERENCES

1. Kolagotla L, Adams W. Ambulatory management of childhood obesity. Obes Res 2004;12(2):275–83. Available at: http://onlinelibrary.wiley.com/doi/10.1038/oby.2004.35/full.
2. Barlow S, Expert Committee. Expert committee recommendations regarding the prevention, assessment, and treatment of child and adolescent overweight and obesity: summary report. Pediatrics 2007;120:S164. Available at: http://pediatrics.aappublications.org/content/120/Supplement_4/S164.full.html.
3. Tanda R, Salsberry P. The impact of the 2007 expert committee recommendations on childhood obesity preventive care in primary care settings in the United States. J Pediatr Health Care 2014;28(3):241–50. Available at: http://www.ncbi.nlm.nih.gov/pmc/articles/PMC3823635/.
4. CDC/NCHS, National Health and Nutrition Examination Survey, Hispanic Health and Nutrition Examination Survey (1982–1984), and National Health Examination Survey (1963–1965 and 1966–1970). See Appendix I, National Health and Nutrition Examination Survey (NHANES). Available at: http://www.cdc.gov/nchs/data/hus/2014/065.pdf. Accessed June 28, 2015.
5. Declining childhood obesity rates: where are we seeing signs of progress? Robert Wood Johnson Foundation; 2015. Available at: http://www.rwjf.org/content/dam/farm/reports/reports/2015/rwjf417749.
6. Peña M-M, Dixon B, Taveras EM. Are you talking to me? The importance of ethnicity and culture in childhood obesity prevention and management. Child Obes 2012;8(1):23–7. Available at: http://www.ncbi.nlm.nih.gov/pmc/articles/PMC3647541/pdf/chi.2011.0109.pdf.
7. Harrison K, Hefner V. Virtually perfect: image retouching and adolescent body image. Media Psychology 2014;17(2):134–53.
8. Available at: http://www.advocatesforyouth.org/publications/publications-a-z/516-adolescent-access-to-confidential-health-services. Accessed June 28, 2015.

9. Jeleleian E, Boergers J, Alday CS, et al. Survey of physician attitudes and practice related to pediatric obesity. Clin Pediatr 2003;42(3):235–45.
10. Clay D, Vignoles VL, Dittmar H. Body image and self-esteem among adolescent girls: testing the influence of sociocultural factors. J Res Adolescence 2005;15(4): 451–77. Available at: http://www.researchgate.net/profile/Helga_Dittmar/publication/227762679_Body_Image_and_SelfEsteem_Among_Adolescent_Girls_Testing_the_Influence_of_Sociocultural_Factors/links/0912f513224e5056db000000.pdf.
11. Spivack J, Swietlik M, Alessandrini E, et al. Primary care providers' knowledge, practices, and perceived barriers to the treatment and prevention of childhood obesity. Obesity 2010;18(7):1341–7. Available at: http://www.researchgate.net/profile/Evaline_Alessandrini/publication/38087044_Primary_care_providers'_knowledge_practices_and_perceived_barriers_to_the_treatment_and_prevention_of_childhood_obesity/links/54db37030cf261ce15cf7db2.pdf.
12. Perez A, Holt N, Gokiert R, et al. Why don't families initiate treatment? A qualitative multicenter study investigating parents' reasons for declining paediatric weight management. Paediatr Child Health 2015;20(4):179–84.
13. Reed VA, Schifferdecker KE, Turco MG. Motivating learning and assessing outcomes in continuing medical education using a personal learning plan. J Contin Educ Health Prof 2012;32(4):287–94.
14. Fryar CD, Gu Q, Ogden CL. Anthropometric reference data for children and adults: United States, 2007–2010. National Center for Health Statistics. Vital Health Stat 2012;11(252):1–40. Available at: http://www.cdc.gov/nchs/data/series/sr_11/sr11_252.pdf.
15. Harris JL, Heard A, Schwartz MB. Older but still vulnerable: all children need protection from unhealthy food marketing. Yale Rudd Center; 2014. Available at: http://www.uconnruddcenter.org/files/Pdfs/Protecting_Older_Children_3_14.pdf.
16. Harris JL, Schwartz MB, Brownwell KD. Marketing foods to children and adolescents: Licensed characters and other promotions on packaged foods in the supermarket. Public Health Nutr 2010;13(3):409–17. Available at: http://journals.cambridge.org/download.php?file=%2FPHN%2FPHN13_03%2FS1368980009991339a.pdf&code=636cc30fa7baa92eead73b8e039e5e6c.
17. Institute of Medicine. Food marketing to children: threat or opportunity? Washington, DC: National Academies Press; 2006. Available at: http://www.nap.edu/openbook.php?record_id=11514&page=R1.
18. Ustjanauskas AE, Harris JL, Schwartz MB. Food and beverage advertising on children's websites. Pediatr Obes 2014;9(5):362–72.
19. Harris JL, Speers SE, Schwartz MB, et al. U.S. food company branded advergames on the internet: children's exposures and effects on snack consumption. J Child Media 2012;6(1):51–68.
20. Bragg MA, Yanamadala S, Roberto CA, et al. Athlete endorsements in food marketing. Pediatrics 2013;132:805–10. Available at: http://pediatrics.aappublications.org/content/early/2013/10/02/peds.2013-0093.full.pdf+html.
21. Dixon H, Scully M, Wakefield M, et al. Parent's responses to nutrient claims and sports celebrity endorsement on energy-dense and nutrient poor foods: an experimental study. Public Health Nutr 2011;14(6):1071–9. Available at: http://journals.cambridge.org/download.php?file=%2FPHN%2FPHN14_06%2FS1368980010003691a.pdf&code=b57445d952d160864786ecfec8f757c2.
22. World Health Organization. A framework for implementing the set of recommendations on the marketing of foods and non-alcoholic beverages to children. 2012. Available at: www.who.int/dietphysicalactivity/framework_marketing_food_to_children/en/. Accessed June 28, 2015.

23. Galbraith-Emami S, Lobstein T. The impact of initiatives to limit the advertising of food and beverage products to children: a systematic review. Obes Rev 2013; 14(2):960–74.

24. Kunckel DL, Castonguay JS, Filer CR. Evaluating industry self-regulation of food marketing to children. Am J Prev Med 2015;49(2):181–7. Available at: http://www.ajpmonline.org/article/S0749-3797(15)00095-1/pdf.

25. Task Force on Community Preventive Services. Physical activity: increasing physical activity through information approaches, behavioral and social approaches, and environmental and policy approaches. The guide to community preventive services. New York; Oxford (England): Task Force on Community Preventive Services; 2005. p. 80–112.

26. Evans WD, Christoffel KK, Mecheles JW, et al. Social marketing as a childhood obesity prevention strategy. Obesity 2010;18(1):s23–6. Available at: http://www.researchgate.net/profile/Doug_Evans/publication/41166460_Social_marketing_as_a_childhood_obesity_prevention_strategy/links/542159ff0cf203f155c65cb1.pdf.

27. Berkowitz JM, Huhman M, Nolin MJ. Did augmenting the VERB campaign advertising in select communities have an effect on awareness, attitudes, and physical activity? Am J Prev Med 2008;34:S257–66. Available at: http://www.ajpmonline.org/article/S0749-3797(08)00252-3/fulltext.

28. Huhman M, Potter LD, Wong FL, et al. Effects of a mass media campaign to increase physical activity among children: year-1 results of the VERB campaign. Pediatrics 2005;116:e277–84. Available at: http://pediatrics.aappublications.org/content/116/2/e277.full.pdf+html.

29. Schuman AJ. Using tech to fight kids' obesity. Contemp Pediatr 2015;32(4):46. Available at: http://contemporarypediatrics.modernmedicine.com/contemporary-pediatrics/news/using-tech-fight-kids-obesity?page=full.

30. Valentin G, Howard AM. Dealing with childhood obesity: passive versus active activity monitoring approaches for engaging individuals in exercise. Biosignals and Biorobotic Conference (BRC). 2013. Rio de Janerio, February 18–20, 2013.

31. Amresh A, Small L. Make your garden grow: designing a physical activity estimation improvement game. Serious Games and Applications for Health (SeGAH). 2014. IEEE 3nd International Conference on SeGAH. Rio de Janeiro, May 14–16, 2014.

32. Appel HB, Huang B, Cole A, et al. Starting the conversation—a childhood obesity knowledge project using an app. Br J Med Med Res 2014;4(7):1526–38. Available at: http://www.ncbi.nlm.nih.gov/pmc/articles/PMC3963698/.

33. Common Sense Media. Social medial, social life: how teens view their digital lives. 2012 & Social Media Today. Facebook demographics revisited—2011 statistic. Available at: http://www.socialmediatoday.com/content/facebook-demographics-revisited-2011-statistics. Accessed June 28, 2015.

34. McCurry M. Systematic Review of Text Messaging as an Intervention for the Treatment of Adolescent Obesity. Nursing Research 2015;64(2).

35. Tucker J, Eisenmann J, Howard K, et al. FitKids360: design, conduct, and outcomes of a stage 2 pediatric obesity program. J Obes 2014;2014:374043. Available at: http://www.hindawi.com/journals/jobe/2014/370403/.

36. Cheng JK, Wen X, Coletti KD, et al. 2-year BMI changes of children referred for multidisciplinary weight management. Int J Pediatr 2014;2014:152586. Available at: http://www.hindawi.com/journals/ijpedi/2014/152586/.

37. Reniscow K, Davis R, Rollnik S. Motivational interviewing for pediatric obesity: conceptual issues and evidence review. J Am Diet Assoc 2006;106(12):2024–33. Available at: http://www.fataids.org/assets/pdf/s0002822306020979.pdf.

38. Whitaker KL, Jarvis MJ, Beeken RJ, et al. Comparing maternal and paternal inter-generational transmission of obesity risk in a large population-based sample. Am J Clin Nutr 2010;91:1560–7. Available at: http://ajcn.nutrition.org/content/91/6/1560.long.
39. Epstein LH, Paluch RA, Wrotniak BH, et al. Cost-effectiveness of family-based group treatment for child and parental obesity. Child Obes 2014;10(2):114–21.
40. Rucker D, Padwal R, Li SK, et al. Long term pharmacotherapy for obesity and overweight: updated meta-analysis. BMJ 2007;335(7631):1194–9. Available at: http://www.bmj.com/content/335/7631/1194.
41. Torgerson JS, Hauptman J, Boldrin MN, et al. Xenical in the Prevention of Diabetes in Obese Subjects (XENDOS) study: a randomized study of orlistat as an adjunct to lifestyle changes for the prevention of type 2 diabetes in obese patients. Diabetes Care 2004;27(1):155–61. Available at: http://care.diabetesjournals.org/content/27/1/155.long.
42. Hanefeld M, Sachse G. The effects of orlistat on body weight and glycemic control in overweight patients with type 2 diabetes: a randomized, placebo controlled trial. Diabetes Obes Metab 2002;4(6):415–23.
43. Hauptman JB, Jeunet FS, Hartmann D. Initial studies in humans with the novel gastrointestinal lipase inhibitor Ro 18-0647(tetrahydrolipstatin). Am J Clin Nutr 1992;55(1 Suppl):309S–13S. Available at: http://ajcn.nutrition.org/content/55/1/309S.long.
44. Miras AD, Le Roux CW. Can medical therapy mimic the clinical efficacy or physiologic effects of bariatric surgery? Int J Obes 2014;28(3):325–33. Available at: http://www.ncbi.nlm.nih.gov/pmc/articles/PMC3372918/.
45. Fox CK, Marlatt KL, Rudser KD, et al. Topiramate for weight reduction in adolescents with severe obesity. Clin Pediatr 2015;54(1):19–24.
46. Kelly AS, Rudser KD, Nathan BM, et al. The effect of glucagon-like peptide-1 receptor agonist therapy on BMI in adolescents with severe obesity: a randomized, placebo-controlled, clinical trial. JAMA Pediatr 2013;167(4):355–60. Available at: http://www.ncbi.nlm.nih.gov/pmc/articles/PMC4010226/pdf/nihms573004.pdf.
47. Inge TH, Krebs KF, Barcia VF, et al. Bariatric surgery for severely overweight adolescents: concerns and recommendations. Pediatrics 2004;11:217–23. Available at: http://www.researchgate.net/profile/Timothy_Kane/publication/8476681_Bariatric_surgery_for_severely_overweight_adolescents_concerns_and_recommendations/links/0912f50b6d58eeca02000000.pdf.

Health Care Systems and National Policy

Role of Leadership in the Obesity Crisis

Jessica Lynn Jones, MD, MSPH*, David Sundwall, MD

KEYWORDS

- Obesity epidemiology • Leadership • Management • Policy

KEY POINTS

- Obesity is a costly epidemic in the United States for children and adults.
- Health care providers, governmental agencies, and nongovernmental agencies have contributing roles in the prevention and treatment of obesity.
- Obesity must be addressed as a public health issue on an individual and population level. Although progress is being made, more work is necessary to reverse the obesity trajectory.

THE OBESITY CHALLENGE: EPIDEMIOLOGY

Obesity is epidemic. Obesity is defined as a body mass index (BMI, calculated as weight in kilograms divided by the square of height in meters) of 30 or higher in adults. The term obesity is new for the pediatric population. Previously, children with excess weight were referred to as being "at risk for overweight" and "overweight."[1] However, current nosology refers to children with a BMI in the 95th percentile or higher for age and sex as obese.[2] Obese children are at risk for becoming obese adults. Obese children have a higher risk of developing hypertension, type 2 diabetes, and hyperlipidemia.[3,4] In adults, obesity is associated with many chronic diseases, including hypertension, type 2 diabetes, gallbladder disease, coronary heart disease, hyperlipidemia, and certain cancers.[5–7] Obese individuals also have a lower life expectancy and increased medical care costs over a lifetime.[7]

In 2009 to 2010, 35% of adults in the United States were obese.[8] Adult obesity significantly increased in the United States from the 1970s to 2000.[9] In 2010, 35% (95% confidence interval [CI], 31.9%–39.2%) of adult men and 36% (95% CI, 34.0%–37.7%) of adult women were obese.[8] This problem extends to the pediatric

Disclosure: The authors have nothing to disclose.
Division of Public Health, Department of Family and Preventive Medicine, University of Utah, 375 Chipeta Way Suite A, Salt Lake City, UT 84108, USA
* Corresponding author.
E-mail address: Jessica.L.Jones@utah.edu

population as well. In 2010, 10% (95% CI, 7.6%–12.3%) of infants aged 0 to 2 years and 17% (95% CI, 15.4%–18.4%) of children aged 2 to 19 years were obese.[10,11]

Between 2011 and 2012, 8% of 2-year-old to 5-year-old children (95% CI, 5.9%–11.6%), 18% of 6-year-old to 11-year-old children (95% CI, 14.5%–21.4%), 21% of 12-year-old to 19-year-old adolescents (95% CI, 17.1%–24.4%), and 35% of adults (95% CI, 32.0%–37.9%) were obese.[12]

The direct costs associated with obesity include diagnosis and treatment. Clinic visits, hospital admissions, nursing home stays, rehabilitation, physical therapy, and medications are all direct obesity costs. Lost productivity, such as wages lost because of illness or death, represent some of the indirect costs associated with obesity.[13] 2008 data suggest that obesity was responsible for a loss of 1.7 to 3.0 million productive years of work for US adults. This finding translates to $390 to 580 billion.[6] Deaths caused by obesity and inactivity are responsible for 14% to 23% of total mortality in the United States. In the 1990s, the health care costs of obesity and inactivity rivaled cigarette smoking, at approximately $47 billion.[13]

Medical costs are higher for obese patients. In 1998, medical spending associated with obesity was $26.8 to $47.5 billion. Health care spending was $732 (35%) greater than that for normal-weight individuals.[14] By 2001, the overall inflation-adjusted per capita medical expenditure was 27% greater than expected. Much of this excess can be attributed to costs associated with increased obesity rates. The 2001 per capita medical expenditure for obese individuals was $1069 (37%) higher than that for normal-weight individuals.[15] By 2006, the per capita medical spending for obesity was $1,429, 42% greater than normal weight (**Table 1**).[16]

The extra medical costs caused by obesity in the United States were approximately $75 billion in 2003 and accounted for 4% to 7% of overall health care expenditures.[14] Health care costs for obesity differ by state. The obesity-attributable fraction (OAF) represents the percentage reduction in medical expenditures that would be realized if all obese individuals were normal weight. The obesity-attributable expenditure (OAE) is the product of OAF and total medical spending. In 2009, Colorado had the lowest OAF (7.0%, 95% CI 5.5%–8.3%), and West Virginia had the highest (11.0%, 95% CI 8.9%–13.1%). Wyoming had the lowest OAE at $203 million (95% CI $164–247 million), and California had the highest with $1.5 billion (95% CI $1.2–$1.8 million).[17]

Current estimates predict that 75% of US adults will be overweight or obese by the year 2020.[18] The projected increase in the cost of obesity is $28 billion per year (85% CI $8–$49 billion) in 2020, and $66 billion per year (95% CI $19–$112 billion) in 2030. A marked improvement in national weight status would improve health, decrease comorbid disease, and significantly reduce health care spending. A 1% reduction in BMI in the United States would avoid 2.1 to 2.4 million new cases of diabetes, 1.4 to 1.7 million new cases of heart disease, and 73,000 to 127,000 new cases of cancer per year.[6]

Table 1
Increase in per capita medical spending for obese adults in the United States for 1998, 2001, and 2006

Year	Difference in Spending Compared with Normal Weight ($) (%)
1998	732 (37.4)[a]
2001	1069 (37.0)[a]
2006	1429 (43)

[a] $P < .05$.
Data from Refs.[14–16]

In December, 2004, the Rosenthal Lecture at the Institute of Medicine directly addressed the US obesity epidemic. A panel of experts summarized this lecture in the subsequently released report, *Perspectives on the Prevention of Childhood Obesity in Children and Youth*. A series of slides presented the scope of this phenomenon using color-coded maps. These maps showed an unrelenting increase in the weight of most Americans, in all states, with an alarming increase in children and youth. Although this finding may not have been news to many in public health and policy circles, it caught the attention of the public, and elevated the national dialogue about what might be done to address this situation. Since that time, myriad activities have been initiated to address what is widely considered the obesity epidemic (**Fig. 1**).

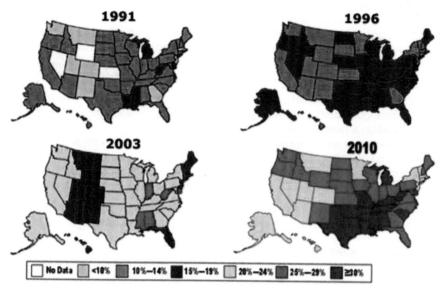

Fig. 1. Prevalence of obesity in the United States. (*From* Centers for Disease Control. Division of Nutrition, Physical Activity, and Obesity. Obesity trends among US adults between 1985 and 2010. Available at: http://www.cdc.gov/obesity/data/prevalence-maps.html.)

RESPONSE TO OBESITY EPIDEMIC

Multiple initiatives have been launched to address the obesity epidemic at all levels of government (federal, states, and local). Health-related foundations, health professional organizations, voluntary health organizations (VHOs), and concerned citizens have also stepped up to play a role to try to stem the rising tide of obesity in America.

Federal Government

The Office of the President

In 2010, President Obama issued a *Presidential Memorandum–Establishing a Task Force on Childhood Obesity*, in which the administration set the ambitious goal of solving the problem of childhood obesity within a generation to allow children to reach adulthood at a healthy weight. The First Lady, Michelle Obama, took on a national public awareness campaign by encouraging involvement from every sector (public, nonprofit, and private), parents, and youth. The purpose of the First Lady's effort was to support and amplify the work of the federal government in improving children's health. The Task Force on Childhood Obesity includes multiple cabinet level appointees, policy experts, and economic advisors.[19] The Let's Move campaign is the First Lady's initiative to combat the epidemic of childhood obesity and encourage a healthy lifestyle. Using a comprehensive, collaborative, and community-oriented approach to address multiple factors that lead to childhood obesity, Let's Move engages multiple sectors of society to affect the health of children. Schools, families, and communities are encouraged to use simple techniques to help children be more active, eat better, and improve their health.[20]

The Office of the Surgeon General

The US Surgeon General is generally recognized as the national spokesperson for promoting healthy behaviors and addressing current public health challenges. The Office of the Surgeon General (OTSG) has promoted awareness of the health consequences of obesity for more than 4 decades, through a series of reports documenting the problem and advocating for policies to promote healthy weight. In 2001, the OTSG published *The Surgeon General's Call To Action To Prevent and Decrease Overweight and Obesity*.[21] This comprehensive document included 5 overarching goals:

1. Promote the recognition of overweight and obesity as major public health problems
2. Help Americans balance healthful eating with regular physical activity to achieve and maintain a healthy weight
3. Identify effective and culturally appropriate interventions to prevent and treat overweight and obesity
4. Encourage environmental changes to prevent overweight and obesity
5. Develop and enhance public-private partnerships to help implement this vision

The most recently appointed US Surgeon General is committed to continuing this focus and improving access to health care services for obese patients.[22]

Department of Health and Human Services

The US Department of Health and Human Services (DHHS) has implemented multiple efforts to address obesity. Public relations campaigns were launched to increase awareness of the scope of the problems related to obesity. Public service announcement have been posted on YouTube.[23] The Physical Activity Guidelines (**Table 2**) for Americans were released in 2008. According to these guidelines, every American should engage in at least 150 minutes (2 hours and 30 minutes) of moderate-intensity activity or 75 minutes (1 hour and 15 minutes) of vigorous-intensity aerobic physical activity or an equivalent combination of moderate-intensity and vigorous-intensity aerobic activity every week. Americans should try to increase their aerobic

Table 2 2008 Physical activity guidelines for Americans	
Key Guidelines for Adults	**Key Guidelines for Children**
• Avoid inactivity Do at least: • 2 h and 30 min/wk of moderate-intensity or • 1 h and 15 min/wk of vigorous-intensity aerobic physical activity or an equivalent combination • Do muscle-strengthening activities on ≥2 d/wk	• 60 min (1 h) or more of physical activity daily ○ Mostly moderate to vigorous-intensity aerobic ○ Vigorous-intensity at least 3 d/wk ○ Muscle strengthening at least 3 d/wk ○ Bone strengthening (weight-bearing) at least 3 d/wk

Data from 2008 Physical Activity Guidelines for Americans. Available at: http://health.gov/paguidelines/guidelines/summary.aspx.

physical activity to 300 minutes (5 hours) a week of moderate-intensity or 150 minutes a week of vigorous-intensity aerobic physical activity or an equivalent combination of moderate-intensity and vigorous-intensity activity. Americans are also encouraged to perform moderate-intensity or high-intensity muscle-strengthening activities that involve all major muscle groups on 2 or more days a week.[24] The Physical Activity Guidelines for American children recommends 60 minutes (1 hour) or more of physical activity daily with a combination of mostly moderate-intensity to vigorous-intensity aerobic activity with vigorous-intensity at least 3 d/wk, Muscle strengthening at least 3 d/wk, and bone strengthening (weight-bearing activity) at least 3 d/wk.[24]

The Office of Disease Prevention and Health Promotion Based in the Office of the Secretary of Health and Human Services, the Office of Disease Prevention and Health Promotion was established to prioritize health goals for the nation through the Healthy People initiatives. The Healthy People goals and objectives are determined by a panel of experts and are organized under topic areas. The goals and objectives and goals are reviewed for progress every 10 years. Leading health indicators are a subset of objectives that highlight high-priority health issues. The Healthy People 2020 objectives in **Table 3** are leading health indicators related to the obesity epidemic in the United States.[25]

These objectives recognize that efforts to change diet and weight must address individual behaviors, as well as the policies and environments that support these behaviors in schools, work sites, health care organizations, and communities. These objectives includes a larger goal of increasing household food security and eliminating hunger.[26]

Centers for Medicare and Medicaid Services obesity management coverage Under the Affordable Care Act (ACA), coverage of specific obesity-related services for Part B Medicare beneficiaries (obesity screening, nutritional assessment, and intensive behavioral therapy for those with a BMI >30) have been expanded when provided in a primary care setting.[27] During his tenure as Administrator of the Centers for Medicare and Medicaid Services (CMS) (2010–2011), Donald Berwick, MD was credited with establishing the policy that public health insurance programs (Medicare and Medicaid) should not just pay for services but achieve the Triple Aim. Specifically, the Triple Aim includes improving the patient experience of care (including quality

Table 3
Healthy people 2020 leading health indicators for obesity

Objective	Description	Goal Prevalence or Intake
Physical activity: 2.4	Increase the proportion of adults who meet the objectives for aerobic physical activity and for muscle-strengthening activity	20.1%
Nutrition and weight status: 9	Reduce the proportion of adults who are obese	30.5%
Nutrition and weight status: 10.4	Reduce the proportion of children and adolescents aged 2–19 y who are considered obese	14.5%
Nutrition and weight status: 15.1	Increase the contribution of total vegetables to the diets of the population aged ≥2 y	1.14 cup per 1000 calories

From USDHHS. Nutrition, Physical Activity, and Obesity. Available at: http://www.healthypeople.gov/2020/leading-health-indicators/2020-lhi-topics/Nutrition-Physical-Activity-and-Obesity. Accessed May 1, 2015.

and satisfaction), improving the health of populations, and reducing the per capita costs of health care. This 3-pronged approach used public health insurance dollars to help achieve public health goals, including obesity prevention and treatment.[28]

The Center for Medicare/Medicaid Innovation The new Center for Medicare/Medicaid Innovation (CMMI) was created under the ACA to develop and test new care models. This strategy includes systems of integrated care and community health. The purpose is to disseminate successful elements of these models through CMS, DHHS, states, local organizations, and industry. As part of this effort, several States Innovation Models (SIMS grants), have been funded to ensure that improvement of population health is appropriately studied and documented. Several state-based CMMI awards directly address obesity.[29]

Medicaid and Children's Health Insurance Program Payment and Access Commission Established in 2010, the Medicaid and Children's Health Insurance Program (CHIP) Payment and Access Commission (MACPAC) is a legislative branch agency that provides policy, data analysis, and recommendations to Congress, the Secretary of the DHHS, and individual states on a wide array of issues affecting Medicaid and the State CHIP. In a 2014 report,[30] MACPAC reviewed population-based strategies to improve the overall health of Medicaid enrollees, including programs to address unhealthy behaviors and obesity.

Public Health Service Agencies

All federal agencies devoted to public health, that is, the National Institutes of Health (NIH), the Centers for Disease Control and Prevention (CDC), the Food and Drug Administration (FDA), the Health Recourses and Services Administration (HRSA), the Agency for Healthcare Research and Quality (AHRQ), the Substance Abuse and Mental Health Services Administration (SAMHSA), and the Indian Health Service, have invested considerable effort and resources into addressing the obesity epidemic in the United States.

National Institutes of Health

The NIH seeks to capitalize on recent scientific discoveries to fund novel efforts toward further understanding the forces contributing to obesity to develop strategies for prevention and treatment. Recognizing that the increase in obesity over the past 30 years has been fueled by a complex interplay of environmental, social, economic, and behavioral factors, within a milieu of genetic susceptibility, the NIH supports a broad spectrum of obesity-related research, including molecular, genetic, behavioral, environmental, clinical, and epidemiologic studies.

Given the importance of the obesity epidemic as a public health problem, and its relevance to the mission of most of the NIH institutes, centers, and offices, the NIH Obesity Research Task Force was established to accelerate progress in obesity research across the NIH. The Task Force is cochaired by the Director of the National Institute of Diabetes and Digestive and Kidney Diseases; the Director of the Eunice Kennedy Shriver National Institute of Child Health and Human Development; and the Director of the National Heart, Lung, and Blood Institute, and includes representatives from most of the research institutes and centers at the NIH.[31]

Centers for Disease Control and Prevention

The CDC established the Division of Nutrition, Physical Activity, and Obesity (DNPAO) to implement policy and environmental strategies to make healthy eating and active living accessible and affordable for everyone. The DNPAO oversees and coordinates multiple activities related to obesity. These activities include public information campaigns about the scope of obesity-related and health-related consequences; data and statistics related to obesity prevalence and trends; a compendium of state initiatives and programs to address obesity; and a robust list of practical resources (social media tools, updated fact sheets, publications) for use by patients and providers. The DNPAO funds grants to state health agencies (state and local) to address obesity (**Table 4**).[32] Other funding mechanisms exist to finance the development and implementation of obesity programs including the Nutrition and Physical Activity Program to Prevent Obesity and Other Chronic Diseases and the Coordinated School Health program.[33]

Agency for Healthcare Research and Quality

AHRQ's mission is to examine and distribute information to make health care safer, of higher quality, more accessible, more equitable, and more affordable. AHRQ is also dedicated to ensuring that evidence is understood and appropriately used.[34] AHRQ has produced several evidence-based reports related to obesity prevention and treatment.[35]

Health Resources and Services Administration

HRSA is an agency within the US DHHS. The HRSA mission is to improve health and achieve health equity through access to quality services, a skilled health workforce, and innovative programs.[36] The HRSA Healthy Weight, Healthy People, Healthy Communities initiative includes several programs that address obesity, focusing on medically underserved communities, including racial and ethnic minority populations (**Table 5**).[37]

Substance Abuse and Mental Health Services Administration

SAMHSA is another agency within the US DHHS. The SAMHSA mission is "to reduce the burden of substance abuse and mental illness."[38] Recognizing obesity as a special challenge for people with mental illness, SAMHSA published a comprehensive document to address these challenges, *Health Promotion Resource Guide: Choosing Evidence-Based Practices for Reducing Obesity and Improving Fitness for People with Serious Mental Illness*.[39]

Table 4 DNPAO funding mechanisms	
Basic Component	**Enhanced Component**
State Public Health Actions is a national program that provides a base level of funding to all 50 states and DC to focus on underlying strategies that address all of these diseases. All states must put into action key strategies in their states including the following DNPAO priority strategies: • Promote the adoption of food service guidelines and nutrition standards, which include sodium • Promote the adoption of physical activity in early child care centers, schools, and work sites	Additional resources are provided to 32 states to enable more intensive interventions and greater health outcomes for these chronic conditions including the following DNPAO priority strategies: • Increase access to healthy foods and beverages • Increase physical activity access and outreach • Increase access to breastfeeding-friendly environments

From Overweight and Obesity. 2015. Available at: www.cdc.gov/obesity/. Accessed June 16, 2015.

Table 5
HRSA Healthy Weight, Healthy People, Healthy Communities programs

Program	Description
Prevention Center for Healthy Weight	A nationwide effort promoting "positive primary care, public health and individual change to reverse the obesity epidemic"
Healthy Weight Collaborative	Teams managed by the prevention center that work to expand obesity treatment and prevention efforts beyond the walls of a clinician's office and into the community
Community health centers	Provide primary health care and use programs (ie, the NIH *We Can!* and Fit-4-Life) to prevent pediatric obesity
Rural health outreach	A grant funding mechanism to develop strategies to address obesity
Maternal and child health	Includes grant funding mechanisms and employer resources to combat obesity
Bright Futures	Guidelines for children, adolescent and women's health

From Healthy Weight, Healthy People, Healthy Communities. Available at: http://www.hrsa.gov/healthyweight/. Accessed June 12, 2015.

US Department of Agriculture

Since 1916, the US Department of Agriculture (USDA) and DHHS have collaborated to provide recommendations for healthy food choices (**Fig. 2**).[40] Every 5 years, the USDA and DHHS review and update the *Dietary Guidelines for Americans*. In 1992, they introduced the Food Guide Pyramid, which was revised to the MyPyramid in 2005. Traditionally, the recommendations were intended for healthy people aged 2 years and older. However, in 2010, the guidelines included recommendations for those at risk for chronic disease. Overall, the *Dietary Guidelines for Americans, 2010*, recommend that people maintain a calorie balance to sustain a healthy weight, which includes avoidance of overeating, and that individuals consume nutrient-dense foods and beverages, avoid excess fat, sodium, sugar, and refined grains, and maximize the intake of fruits, vegetables, whole grains, reduced fat milk products, seafood, lean meat and poultry, eggs, legumes, nuts, and seeds.[25]

Based on the 2010 guidelines, the USDA Center for Nutrition Policy and Promotion launched the MyPlate initiative.[41] This revised version of the previous food pyramids encourages people to think about food choices and proportions with a simple visual cue. Revisions to the MyPlate Web site (www.ChooseMyPlate.gov) include an interactive and personalized tool for tracking diet and physical activity, activities for children aged 8 to 12 years, and initiatives for college campuses.[42,43] The uptake and acceptance of MyPlate has been good. Recent surveys[44] indicate that most dieticians (75%) use MyPlate resources and 61% of consumers are aware of the MyPlate initiative.

Food and Drug Administration

The FDA is responsible for ensuring the safety and efficacy of foods, drugs, cosmetics, medical devices, vaccinations, biological products, and laboratory tests. The FDA is at the forefront of the government's efforts to protect the public's health. On December 1, 2015, the FDA implemented the first federal nutrition-labeling mandate in more than 2 decades. This mandate preempts existing local or state laws. This regulation requires food establishments to clearly show the calorie count of standard menu items. Although studies have not identified a statistically significant change in calorie consumption from menu labeling, it is believed that on a population level, even a small

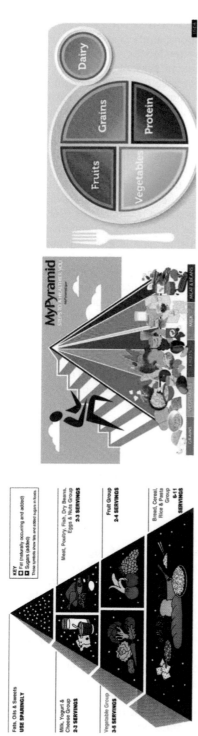

Fig. 2. Icons associated with dietary guidelines for Americans 1992–2011. (*From* US Department of Agriculture. National Agricultural Library: Food and Nutrition Information Center. Available at: http://fnic.nal.usda.gov/.)

reduction in caloric intake will reduce the likelihood of chronic diseases such obesity and diabetes.[45]

The FDA plays another important role in addressing the obesity epidemic through review of drugs and devices intended for weight loss. Although there is considerable interest in having such products available to assist in the clinical care of obese patients, there is also considerable cause for concern in approving and promoting medications used for these purposes. A widely known example is the drug combination fenfluramine/phentermine (fen-phen). Fenfluramine was shown to cause potentially fatal pulmonary hypertension and heart valve problems, which led to its withdrawal from the market. However, phentermine was not found to be harmful when used as a single agent. Phentermine is still used as an anorectic agent to help with weight loss.

Although many drugs have been submitted to the FDA for review and approval, most were found lacking in some aspects of safety or efficacy.[46] Three drugs are approved for clinical use. Lorcaserin hydrochloride (Belviq) is a serotonin 2C receptor agonist that may promote early satiety. Phentermine with topiramate (Qysmia) has also been approved. Phentermine is a central nervous system stimulant and topiramate is an antiseizure medication. Bupropion with naltrexone (Contrave)is another combination drug that is available. Bupropion is an antidepressant and naltrexone blocks the effects of narcotics and alcohol.[47]

Although these drugs have gained FDA approval, none has gained broad usage. Medicare, most state Medicaid programs, and some commercial insurers do not pay for the drugs. Providers and patients are cautious about safety because of adverse outcomes with previous weight loss drugs. Furthermore, weight loss is often modest with the use of these medications.[48]

FDA-regulated medical devices have also played a role in treating obesity. There are 4 FDA-approved devices on the market designed to treat obesity:

- Lap-Band gastric banding system
- Realize gastric band
- The Maestro rechargeable system
- ReShape integrated dual balloon system

These devices are clinically indicated only for patients with at least 1 comorbidity who have failed to lose weight with dedicated lifestyle changes.[49]

State Governments

Many states have enacted a variety of legislative and regulatory policies in response to increasing obesity rates. From 2001 to 2010, more than 600 state-level obesity-specific bills were proposed, and almost 100 were enacted. These bills focused on initiatives such as taskforce augmentation, health care improvements, school interventions, and community engagement.[50] Between 2010 and 2013, 81 of 487 (16%) bills for adult obesity prevention were enacted in the United States. More bills focused on physical activity and diet (37% vs 13%). Food and beverage tax bills were least likely to be adopted. Infrastructure and building bills were adopted most frequently (42%).[51] States receiving funding for obesity programs enacted significantly more obesity bills compared with nonfunded states (2.6 per state vs 1.2 per state). CDC-funded states passed legislative bills to combat obesity at the highest rates. CDC-funded states passed an average of 3.3 bills per state, whereas unfunded states passed an average of 1.4 bills.[33]

Private Foundations

Independent private foundations offer financial support to many different causes. Companies, citizens, governments, or nongovernmental organizations can create foundations. There are a few notable foundations contributing to the fight against obesity.

Robert Wood Johnson Foundation

As the largest philanthropic organization in the United States, the mission of the Robert Wood Johnson Foundation (RWJF) is to improve the health and health care of all Americans. A primary focus of the RWJF is childhood obesity.[52] Building on a $500 million commitment made in 2007, the RWJF recently announced[53] an additional $500 million for obesity-related projects to ensure that all children in the United States grow up at a healthy weight.

Aetna Foundation

The mission of the Aetna Foundation is to promote wellness, health, and access to high-quality health care for everyone. The Aetna Foundation offers grants focusing on issues that improve health and the health care system. One of the focus areas for funding is healthy eating and active living to create a better understanding of the root causes of the obesity epidemic.[54]

W.K. Kellogg Foundation

The Kellogg Foundation focuses on childhood development. One of their 3 core strategic goals (Healthy Kids) supports efforts to reduce childhood obesity.[55]

Dr Robert C. and Veronica Atkins Foundation

The Atkins Foundation supports investigations on the roles of metabolism and nutrition in disease prevention and management. This foundation funds obesity-focused independent research, endows academic chair positions dedicated to the study of obesity, and funds centers for excellence in obesity management.[56]

New Balance Foundation

Focusing on childhood obesity, the mission of the New Balance Foundation is to support charitable organizations whose humanitarian efforts work for the betterment of children and communities.[57]

Voluntary Health Organizations

VHOs are not-for-profit groups providing public education and advocacy on behalf of patients suffering from specific illnesses or conditions. VHOs provide patient support and contribute to research, prevention efforts, treatments, and health care access. Several large VHOs devote considerable attention to addressing the obesity epidemic. The following are a few examples:

American Diabetes Association

The American Diabetes Association (ADA) (www.ada.org) publishes hundreds of articles related to obesity that cover a broad range of topics (eg, children in day care, nursing mothers, family dynamics). The ADA is an outstanding resource that not only focuses on obesity and its relationship with diabetes but also obesity prevention, treatment, and epidemiology. Although most of the publications are intended for a general audience, there are also scientific articles useful for health professionals.[58]

American Heart Association

The American Heart Association (AHA) (www.americanheart.org) also publishes hundreds of articles related to obesity and its association with heart disease. The AHA has well-researched information about physical activity, nutrition, and heart disease, along with useful epidemiologic data and information about the role of health disparities.[58]

American Cancer Society

The American Cancer Society (http://www.cancer.org/) publishes articles describing the association between obesity and certain cancers (colon, breast, and prostate). Other articles cover general issues such as nutrition and the association of greater risk of cancer with physical inactivity.[59]

Health Care and Hospital Systems

Many health care systems have developed their own programs to combat the obesity epidemic. One notable example is the Intermountain Healthcare system. Intermountain Healthcare is an internationally recognized, not-for-profit health care organization located in Utah and southeastern Idaho[60] known for low-cost, integrated health care delivery.

Intermountain Healthcare published its *Lifestyle and Weight Management* (LWM) *Care Process Model* (CPM) in 2013.[61] The LWM/CPM is part of a larger organizational wellness and health promotion program, called LiVe Well. A multidisciplinary team of physicians and other health care providers created the LWM/CPM. Rather than focusing on weight management alone, this model encompasses lifestyle behaviors that contribute to overall health and well-being. These behaviors are generally the same behaviors that support healthy weight management. The CPM moves beyond what to do; it focuses on why it matters and how to be successful. Its purpose is to summarize and promote evidence-based approaches to lifestyle and weight management and to facilitate implementation in routine primary care. The emphasis is on improved health and well-being, not just weight loss. The LWM/CPM also addresses sedentary activity, nutrition and healthy eating habits, sleep, stress, social support, and mental health. It concludes with weight management strategies, including indications for bariatric surgery and the risks and benefits of weight loss medications. The model is dependent on team-based care. This team includes physicians, dietitians, physical therapists, mental health professionals, sleep specialists, and other allied health professionals.

Grass Roots Leadership and Change from the Ground Up: Life in Primary Care Practices

Primary care providers are perhaps in the best position to encourage individual behavioral change in regard to obesity. However, most fail to do so. Only 30% and 42% of overweight and obese patients, respectively, report that their primary care provider advised them to lose weight within the past year.[62,63] Only about 10% of obese patients have the diagnosis of obesity documented in their clinical record. This finding is important because patients carrying a documented diagnosis of obesity are more likely to receive formal dietary counseling.[64] The American College of Preventive Medicine and the American Medical Association recommend weight management counseling for all obese patients, both adults and children.[65,66] Obese individuals whose provider advised weight loss are more likely to try to lose weight compared with those not counseled.[63] Most overweight and obese patients want their physician to help them with their weight and trust their doctor to help.[67] In general, most patients are comfortable discussing weight issues and believe that weight loss is important.[67]

Negative provider bias against obese patients, lack of adequate compensation, and lack of adequate training in behavior counseling conspire to limit counseling in individual primary care practices.[64,68] Obesity counseling merits a specific, individual visit that is not combined with other conditions. Providers (defined as a physician specializing in family, internal, geriatric, or pediatric medicine, or a nurse practitioner, clinical nurse specialist, or physician assistant)[69] can be compensated for an assessment of eligibility and subsequent behavioral therapy. New policies with the ACA and CMS specifically aim to improve compensation and training.[70] New CMS policy assumes that providers are able effectively to provide behavioral counseling for weight loss in the context of a traditional 15-minute clinic visit. However, undergraduate and graduate medical education accreditation bodies do not mandate specific behavioral counseling guidelines for medical students and residents.[71,72]

Many providers are not comfortable in their ability to prescribe effective weight loss regimens to their obese patients.[73–77] The 5A model (ask, advise, assess, assist, and arrange) for obesity counseling is 1 simple tool that increases odds of patient motivation and intention for behavior changes toward weight improvement.[78] Motivational interviewing is another simple and effective tool that providers can use for effective behavioral change and obesity counseling.[79] Healthy Eating Vital Signs (HEVS) is a concise screening tool to identify key eating behaviors associated with excessive weight.[80,81] HEVS focuses on restaurant and fast food consumption, large portion size, sugar-sweetened beverage consumption, fruit and vegetable consumption, and healthy breakfast consumption. These specific behaviors are amenable to brief clinic-based counseling for prevention and treatment of obesity.[82] Two valid and reliable questionnaires exist to assess physical activity in adults: the Rapid Assessment of Physical Activity[83] and the Physical Activity Assessment Tool 3.[84]

Physical Activity Vital Sign (PAVS) uses 2 questions to assess moderate to vigorous physical activity levels: (1) How many days during the past week have you performed physical activity where your heart beats faster and your breathing is harder than normal for 30 minutes or more? (2) How many days in a typical week do you perform activity such as this? The responses are reported in a format similar to blood pressure, that is, days during past week over days in typical week. The responses yield a PAVS score ranging from a minimum of 0/0 to a maximum of 7/7. PAVS takes less than 30 seconds to administer and score. It provides valuable longitudinal information regarding physical activity that can be used in the context of provider-patient conversations about weight managment.[85]

MEDICAL MANAGEMENT OF OBESITY: MERGING INDIVIDUALS AND SYSTEMS

The American Medical Association, Council of the Obesity Society, and American Association of Clinical Endocrinologists classify obesity as a chronic disease. The paradigm for treatment of obesity is founded on lifestyle modification. Pharmacotherapy and surgery are available adjuncts for selected patients (**Fig. 3**).

Lifestyle Modification

Lifestyle modifications (see the articles elsewhere in this issue) include dietary modifications and caloric restriction, augmenting physical activity, and providing techniques for self-monitoring and sustained behavioral change. Caloric restriction is a priority for weight loss, whereas physical activity is required for maintenance of lost weight.[86] Pharmacotherapy (see article elsewhere in this issue) is available as an adjunct to lifestyle modifications in selected patients. The FDA regulates the availability of prescription and over-the-counter medications in the United States. In general, if individuals

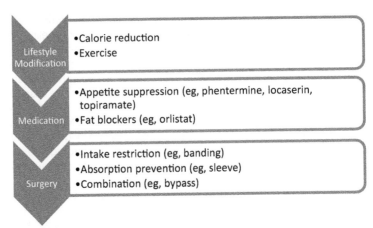

Fig. 3. Paradigm for treating obesity. (*Data from* Kushner RF. Weight loss strategies for treatment of obesity. Prog Cardiovasc Dis 2014;56(4):465–72; and Kakkar AK, Dahiya N. Drug treatment of obesity: current status and future prospects. Eur J Intern Med 2015;26(2):89–4.)

have not lost 5% of their body weight after 3 months of pharmacotherapy, the medication should be discontinued.[86] When lifestyle modification and pharmacotherapy fail, bariatric surgery procedures are available. Candidates for bariatric surgery include those with BMI 40 or higher or BMI 35 or higher and other comorbidities, that is, hypertension, dyslipidemia, and osteoarthritis. Three bariatric surgery approaches are most widely used: restrictive (ie, banding) procedures, malabsorptive (ie, bypass) procedures, and combined approaches. Restrictive or banding procedures decrease the size of the gastric opening. Malabsorptive procedures reroute the gastrointestinal system to reduce the digestion of nutrients. Bariatric procedures also alter gastrointestinal hormone homeostasis and adipose metabolism to reduce weight.[86]

FUTURE OPPORTUNITIES
Research

There are multiple funding opportunities for investigators dedicated to managing the obesity epidemic. Many national and regional nongovernmental organizations and foundations invest considerable financial resources in obesity-related projects. These agencies and organizations are creating, augmenting, evaluating, and promoting strategies to prevent and treat obesity in various populations.

Policy

Creating and enacting a bill is the first step to initiating change in public health law. Many public health laws are inconsistent, ambiguous, and dated. New obesity legislation should reflect the duty of government to promote population's health and well-being, provide authorities with the autonomy to regulate health and security, and restrain government from limiting individual authority, liberty, and privacy.[87]

Providers should be informed about policies and have the knowledge and influence to improve population health.[88] Three steps to the policy process include (1) problem recognition, (2) identification of policies to solve the problem, and (3) establishment of a political environment to successfully adopt proposed policies. Activities to engage this 3-domain process include accessing the target population, collaborating with stakeholders (ie, legislators), and gathering support.[88]

SUMMARY

With a predominant culture of inactivity and caloric excess, obesity is epidemic in the United States. This chronic disease is costly, physically and financially. Obesity increases the risk of many chronic diseases and premature death. It greatly increases medical expenditure as well. Although obesity can be addressed on an individual basis, it is largely recognized as a public health issue. The broad response to obesity includes efforts from medical providers, local and federal governments, and nongovernmental agencies. Working together to create individual change in the examination room and policy change in halls of legislation will stem the rising tide of obesity in the United States.

ACKNOWLEDGMENTS

The authors would like to acknowledge Liz Joy, MD, MPH of Intermountain Healthcare for her contributions to this article.

REFERENCES

1. Barlow SE, Dietz WH. Obesity evaluation and treatment: expert committee recommendations. The Maternal and Child Health Bureau, Health Resources and Services Administration and the Department of Health and Human Services. Pediatrics 1998;102(3):E29.
2. Barlow SE, Expert C. Expert committee recommendations regarding the prevention, assessment, and treatment of child and adolescent overweight and obesity: summary report. Pediatrics 2007;120(Suppl 4):S164–92.
3. Serdula MK, Ivery D, Coates RJ, et al. Do obese children become obese adults? A review of the literature. Prev Med 1993;22(2):167–77.
4. Freedman DS, Mei Z, Srinivasan SR, et al. Cardiovascular risk factors and excess adiposity among overweight children and adolescents: the Bogalusa Heart Study. J Pediatr 2007;150(1):12–7.e2.
5. Must A, Spadano J, Coakley EH, et al. The disease burden associated with overweight and obesity. JAMA 1999;282(16):1523–9.
6. Wang YC, McPherson K, Marsh T, et al. Health and economic burden of the projected obesity trends in the USA and the UK. Lancet 2011;378(9793):815–25.
7. Thompson D, Edelsberg J, Colditz GA, et al. Lifetime health and economic consequences of obesity. Arch Intern Med 1999;159(18):2177–83.
8. Flegal KM, Carroll MD, Kit BK, et al. Prevalence of obesity and trends in the distribution of body mass index among US adults, 1999-2010. JAMA 2012;307(5): 491–7.
9. Hedley AA, Ogden CL, Johnson CL, et al. Prevalence of overweight and obesity among US children, adolescents, and adults, 1999-2002. JAMA 2004;291(23): 2847–50.
10. Ogden CL, Carroll MD, Curtin LR, et al. Prevalence of high body mass index in US children and adolescents, 2007-2008. JAMA 2010;303(3):242–9.
11. Ogden CL, Carroll MD, Kit BK, et al. Prevalence of obesity and trends in body mass index among US children and adolescents, 1999-2010. JAMA 2012; 307(5):483–90.
12. Ogden CL, Carroll MD, Flegal KM. Prevalence of obesity in the United States. JAMA 2014;312(2):189–90.
13. Colditz GA. Economic costs of obesity and inactivity. Med Sci Sports Exerc 1999; 31(11 Suppl):S663–7.

14. Finkelstein EA, Fiebelkorn IC, Wang G. National medical spending attributable to overweight and obesity: how much, and who's paying? Health Aff (Millwood) 2003;(Suppl Web Exclusives):W3-W219–W-326.
15. Thorpe KE, Florence CS, Howard DH, et al. The impact of obesity on rising medical spending. Health Aff (Millwood) 2004;(Suppl Web Exclusives):W4-W480–486.
16. Finkelstein EA, Trogdon JG, Cohen JW, et al. Annual medical spending attributable to obesity: payer-and service-specific estimates. Health Aff (Millwood) 2009;28(5):w822–31.
17. Trogdon JG, Finkelstein EA, Feagan CW, et al. State- and payer-specific estimates of annual medical expenditures attributable to obesity. Obesity (Silver Spring) 2012;20(1):214–20.
18. Sassi F. Obesity and the economics of prevention: fit not fat. 2010. Available at: http://www.oecd.org/els/health-systems/46044572.pdf2015. Accessed June 15, 2015.
19. Presidential Memorandum: Establishing a Task Force on Childhood Obesity. 2010. Available at: https://www.whitehouse.gov/the-press-office/presidential-memorandum-establishing-a-task-force-childhood-obesity. Accessed June 16, 2015.
20. First Lady Michelle Obama Launches Let's Move: America's Move to Raise a Healthier Generation of Kids. 2010. Available at: https://www.whitehouse.gov/the-press-office/first-lady-michelle-obama-launches-lets-move-americas-move-raise-a-healthier-genera. Accessed June 16, 2015.
21. The Surgeon General's Call to Action to Prevent and Decrease Overweight and Obesity. 2001. Available at: http://www.ncbi.nlm.nih.gov/books/NBK44206/. Accessed June 16, 2016.
22. US Surgeon General is Committed to Addressing Obesity. 2014. Available at: www.obesity.org/news-center/us-surgeon-general-committed-to-addressing-obesity.htm. Accessed June 16, 2016.
23. PlowShareGroup. Sandbags. YouTube; 2012.
24. 2008 Physical Activity Guidelines for Americans In: USDHHS, editor; 2008. Available at: http://health.gov/paguidelines/guidelines/summary.aspx.
25. USDHHS. Nutrition, Physical Activity, and Obesity. Available at: http://www.healthypeople.gov/2020/leading-health-indicators/2020-lhi-topics/Nutrition-Physical-Activity-and-Obesity. Accessed May 1, 2015.
26. Nutrition and Weight Status. Available at: www.healthypeople.gov/2020/topics-objectives/topic/nutrition-and-weight-status. Accessed June 16, 2016.
27. Your Medicare Coverage. Available at: http://www.medicare.gov/coverage/obesity-screening-and-counseling.html Accessed June 26, 2015.
28. Berwick DM, Nolan TW, Whittington J. The triple aim: care, health, and cost. Health Aff (Millwood) 2008;27(3):759–69.
29. Innovation Models. Available at: innovation.cms.gov/initiatives/index.html#views=models. Accessed June 16, 2016.
30. Medicaid and Population Health. 2014. Available at: www.macpac.gov/publication/ch-3-medicaid-and-population-health/. Accessed June 16, 2015.
31. About NIH Obesity Research. 2015. Available at: www.obesityresearch.nih.gov/about/about.aspx. Accessed June 16, 2015.
32. Overweight and Obesity. 2015. Available at: www.cdc.gov/obesity/. Accessed June 16, 2015.
33. Hersey J, Lynch C, Williams-Piehota P, et al. The association between funding for statewide programs and enactment of obesity legislation. J Nutr Educ Behav 2010;42(1):51–6.

34. About AHRQ. 2015. Available at: http://www.ahrq.gov/cpi/about/index.html. Accessed June 12, 2015.
35. Evidence-based Practice Center Reports Topic Index: A-Z. Available at: http://www.ahrq.gov/research/findings/evidence-based-reports/a-z/index.html#Otopics. Accessed June 10, 2015.
36. About HRSA. Available at: http://www.hrsa.gov/about/index.html. Accessed June 12, 2015.
37. Healthy Weight, Healthy People, Healthy Communities. Available at: http://www.hrsa.gov/healthyweight/. Accessed June 12, 2015.
38. About Us. Available at: http://www.samhsa.gov/about-us. Accessed June 12, 2015.
39. Health promotion resource guide: choosing evidence-based practices for reducing obesity and improving fitness for people with serious mental illness. SAMHSA-HRSA Center for Integrated Health Solutions; 2014. Available at: http://www.integration.samhsa.gov/health-wellness/Health_Promotion_Guide.pdf.
40. Urakpa FO, Moeckly BG, Fulfod LD, et al. Awareness and use of MyPlate guidelines in making food choices. Procedia Food Sci 2013;2:180–6.
41. Levine E, Abbatangelo-Gray J, Mobley AR, et al. Evaluating MyPlate: an expanded framework using traditional and nontraditional metrics for assessing health communication campaigns. J Nutr Educ Behav 2012;44(4):S2–12.
42. Post RE, Mainous AG 3rd, Gregorie SH, et al. The influence of physician acknowledgment of patients' weight status on patient perceptions of overweight and obesity in the United States. Arch Intern Med 2011;171(4):316–21.
43. Post RC, Maniscalco S, Herrup M, et al. What's new on MyPlate? A new message, redesigned web site, and SuperTracker debut. J Acad Nutr Diet 2012;112(1):18–22.
44. Haven J, Maniscalco S, Bard S, et al. MyPlate myths debunked. J Acad Nutr Diet 2014;114(5):674–5.
45. Larner L. New Health Policy Brief: The FDA's Menu-Labeling Rule Health Affairs 2015. Available at: http://healthaffairs.org/blog/2015/06/29/new-health-policy-brief-the-fdas-menu-labeling-rule/.
46. Colman E. Food and Drug Administration's obesity drug guidance document: a short history. Circulation 2012;125(17):2156–64.
47. New Obesity Drug, Contrave, Gets FDA Approval. Health. 2014.
48. Pollack A. New drug to treat obesity gains approval by FDA. New York Times 2014.
49. Obesity Treatment Devices. 2015. Available at: http://www.fda.gov/Medical Devices/ProductsandMedicalProcedures/ObesityDevices/default.htm. Accessed June 26, 2015.
50. Lankford T, Hardman D, Dankmeyer C, et al. Analysis of state obesity legislation from 2001 to 2010. J Public Health Manag Pract 2013;19(3 Suppl 1):S114–8.
51. Donaldson EA, Cohen JE, Villanti AC, et al. Patterns and predictors of state adult obesity prevention legislation enactment in US states: 2010-2013. Prev Med 2015;74:117–22.
52. Childhood Obesity. Available at: http://www.rwjf.org/en/our-topics/topics/childhood-obesity.html. Accessed May 19, 2015.
53. Robert Wood Johnson Foundation Doubles Its Commitment to Helping All Children Grow Up at a Healthy Weight. 2015. Available at: www.rwjf.org/en/library/articles-and-news/2015/02/rwjf_doubles_commitment_to_healthy_weight_for_children.html. Accessed July 1, 2015.

54. Healthy Eating and Active Living. Available at: http://www.aetna-foundation.org/foundation/aetna-foundation-programs/obesity/index.html. Accessed May 19, 2015.

55. What We Do. Available at: https://www.wkkf.org/what-we-do/overview. Accessed May 19, 2015.

56. About. Available at: http://www.atkinsfoundation.org/about. Accessed May 19, 2015.

57. The New Balance Foundation. Available at: http://www.newbalancefoundation.org/. Accessed May 19, 2015.

58. Available at: www.heart.org/HEARTORG/search/searchResults.jsp?_dyncharset=ISO-8859-1&;q=obesity. Accessed June 26, 2015.

59. Available at: www.cancer.org/search/index?QueryText=obesity&;Page=1. Accessed June 26, 2015.

60. Welcome to Intermountain Healthcare. Available at: http://intermountainhealthcare.org/Pages/home.aspx. Accessed July 2, 2015.

61. Care Process Model 2013.

62. Sciamanna CN, Tate DF, Lang W, et al. Who reports receiving advice to lose weight? Results from a multistate survey. Arch Intern Med 2000;160(15):2334–9.

63. Galuska DA, Will JC, Serdula MK, et al. Are health care professionals advising obese patients to lose weight? JAMA 1999;282(16):1576–8.

64. Bleich SN, Pickett-Blakely O, Cooper LA. Physician practice patterns of obesity diagnosis and weight-related counseling. Patient Educ Couns 2011;82(1):123–9.

65. Nawaz H, Katz DL. American College of Preventive Medicine Practice Policy statement. Weight management counseling of overweight adults. Am J Prev Med 2001;21(1):73–8.

66. Rao G. Childhood obesity: highlights of AMA Expert Committee recommendations. Am Fam Physician 2008;78(1):56–63.

67. Potter MB, Vu JD, Croughan-Minihane M. Weight management: what patients want from their primary care physicians. J Fam Pract 2001;50(6):513–8.

68. Lyznicki JM, Young DC, Riggs JA, et al, Council on Scientific Affairs AMA. Obesity: assessment and management in primary care. Am Fam Physician 2001;63(11):2185–96.

69. Centers for Disease Control and Prevention (CDC). Vital signs: state-specific obesity prevalence among adults—United States, 2009. MMWR Morb Mortal Wkly Rep 2010;59(30):951–5.

70. CMS. Decision Memo for Intensive Behavioral Therapy for Obesity2011. Available at: http://www.cms.gov/medicare-coverage-database/details/nca-decision-memo.aspx?&NcaName=Intensive%20Behavioral%20Therapy%20for%20Obesity&bc=ACAAAAAAIAAA&NCAId=253&. Accessed April 15, 2015.

71. Liaison Committee on Medical Education. Functions and structure of a medical school. In: Liaison Committee on Medical Education, editor. Washington, DC: Standards for accreditation of medical education programs leading to the MD Degree; 2012. p. 8–10.

72. Liaison Committee on Medical Education/Committee on Accreditation of Canadian Medical Schools. Medical Education Database 2012-2013. Washington, DC: LCME/CACMS; 2012.

73. Adimoolam V, Charney P. Identification and management of overweight and obesity by internal medicine residents: Christopher B. Ruser, Lisa Sanders et al. J Gen Intern Med 2006;21(10):1128.

74. Davis NJ, Shishodia H, Taqui B, et al. Resident physician attitudes and competence about obesity treatment: need for improved education. Med Educ Online 2008;13:5.

75. Blalock SJ, Norton LL, Patel RA, et al. Development and assessment of a short instrument for assessing dietary intakes of calcium and vitamin D. J Am Pharm Assoc (2003) 2003;43(6):685–93.
76. Forman-Hoffman V, Little A, Wahls T. Barriers to obesity management: a pilot study of primary care clinicians. BMC Fam Pract 2006;7:35.
77. Kushner RF. Barriers to providing nutrition counseling by physicians: a survey of primary care practitioners. Prev Med 1995;24(6):546–52.
78. Jay M, Gillespie C, Schlair S, et al. Physicians' use of the 5As in counseling obese patients: is the quality of counseling associated with patients' motivation and intention to lose weight? BMC Health Serv Res 2010;10:159.
79. Burton AM, Agne AA, Lehr SM, et al. Training residents in obesity counseling: incorporating principles of motivational interviewing to enhance patient centeredness. J Grad Med Educ 2011;3(3):408–11.
80. Greenwood JLJ, Arguello D, Lin J, et al. Healthy Eating Vital Sign (HEVS): a new assessment tool for eating behaviors. ISRN Obes 2012;2012:7.
81. Greenwood JLJ, Murtaugh MA, Omura EM, et al. Creating a clinical screening questionnaire for eating behaviors associated with overweight and obesity. J Am Board Fam Med 2008;21(6):539–48.
82. Greenwood JLJ, Stanford JB. Preventing or improving obesity by addressing specific eating patterns. J Am Board Fam Med 2008;21:135–40.
83. Topolski TD, LoGerfo J, Patrick DL, et al. The Rapid Assessment of Physical Activity (RAPA) among older adults. Prev Chronic Dis 2006;3(4):A118.
84. Meriwether RA, McMahon PM, Islam N, et al. Physical activity assessment: validation of a clinical assessment tool. Am J Prev Med 2006;31(6):484–91.
85. Greenwood JLJ, Joy EA, Stanford JB. The physical activity vital sign: a primary care tool to guide counseling for obesity. J Phys Act Health 2010;7(5):571–6.
86. Kushner RF. Weight loss strategies for treatment of obesity. Prog Cardiovasc Dis 2014;56(4):465–72.
87. Gostin LO. Public health law reform. Am J Public Health 2001;91(9):1365–8.
88. IOM. For the Public's Health: Revitalizing Law and Policy to Meet New Challenges. 2011. Available at: https://www.iom.edu/Reports/2011/For-the-Publics-Health-Revitalizing-Law-and-Policy-to-Meet-New-Challenges.aspx. Accessed May 1, 2015.

Obesity Prevention and Screening

Eleanor R. Mackey, PhD[a],*, Alexandra Olson, BA[b], Marc DiFazio, MD[c],
Omni Cassidy, MS[d]

KEYWORDS

- Obesity • Screening • Prevention • Development

KEY POINTS

- Screen for weight status at every primary care visit. Screening tools vary by age.
- Communicate appropriately and effectively with patients to maximize the success of prevention efforts. Motivational interviewing promotes patient willingness to engage in behavioral change.
- Prevention recommendations vary by age and stage of development, and cultural context is critical. Core behaviors include dietary intake, physical activity, and sleep.

INTRODUCTION

Obesity is one of the most significant public health crises of our time. Between 5% and 10% of US health care costs are spent on the treatment of overweight, obesity, and associated comorbidities.[1] Obesity in adults is associated with increased risk for cardiovascular, metabolic disease, and cancer.[2] Overweight and obesity are also occurring in high rates in younger populations. In obese children, in addition to higher risk for cardiovascular and metabolic disease, there are also social and psychological difficulties,[3] such that the quality of life of obese youth has been compared with those with cancer.[4] Obese youth are likely to be overweight and obese adults, thus conferring a lifetime of risk for medical and psychosocial difficulties.[5,6] Obesity has a high

Disclosures: The authors have no commercial or financial conflicts of interest or any funding sources to disclose.
[a] Department of Psychology and Behavioral Health, Children's National Health System, 111 Michigan Avenue Northwest, Washington, DC 20010, USA; [b] Children's National Health System, Center for Translational Science, 111 Michigan Avenue Northwest, Washington, DC 20010, USA; [c] Department of Neurology, Children's National Health System, 9850 Key West Avenue, 4th Floor, Rockville, MD 20850, USA; [d] Department of Medical and Clinical Psychology, Uniformed Services University of the Health Sciences, 4301 Jones Bridge Road, Bethesda, MD 20814, USA
* Corresponding author.
E-mail address: emackey@childrensnational.org

Prim Care Clin Office Pract 43 (2016) 39–51
http://dx.doi.org/10.1016/j.pop.2015.08.009
0095-4543/16/$ – see front matter © 2016 Elsevier Inc. All rights reserved.

individual and societal cost. For example, absenteeism is increased for obese children[7] and adults because of missed school, missed work, and increased health care use.[8,9]

SCREENING AND PREVENTION

The lack of broadly effective treatments for obesity[10] highlights the importance of efficacious screening and prevention.[11,12] From a population health perspective, everyone should be screened for obesity and obesity risk, and targeted prevention applied. The risk for becoming obese is present across at all ages. However, prevention targets differ by age group and cultural context so this must also be taken into account. Primary care practices should be aware of contextual considerations by age group and culture, have ready access to available screening tools, and be comfortable with approaches to prevention.

INFANTS (BIRTH–12 MONTHS), TODDLERS (1–3 YEARS), AND PRESCHOOLERS (3–5 YEARS)

There is a unique opportunity for obesity prevention at very young ages.[13] The first 4 to 6 months of life (when birth weight typically doubles) can set the foundation for future weight trajectories. Infants who have excess fat at birth or who rapidly gain weight in the first 6 months of life are at risk for adult obesity.[14–16] Interventions to promote appropriate weight gain during the first 6 months of life have a substantial impact on future weight trajectories.

The toddler and preschool years also set the foundation for eating behaviors, physical activity patterns, and weight trajectories.[17] Timing of the introduction of solid foods, parental modeling of appropriate eating behaviors, sound sleep hygiene habits, limits on screen time, and encouragement of physical activity all develop during this time period.[18] These are critical target behaviors to help prevent the onset of obesity.

Screening Tools

World Health Organization (WHO) measurements are used to classify obesity for infancy through preschool. WHO standards have shorter growth measurement intervals and provide the most accuracy for the rapid growth period between infancy and early childhood.[19] Obese infants are greater than or equal to the 95th percentile for weight for recumbent length.[20] As children age, standing height is included and clinicians typically switch to US Centers for Disease Control and Prevention (CDC) growth charts for weight-for-stature measurements for toddlers and preschoolers.[20]

The 95th percentile of the sex-specific CDC growth charts for body mass index (BMI) for age defines obesity in toddlers and preschoolers.[21] Weight and recumbent length measurements are an established element of routine well-child care. All measurements should be taken and recorded in a standard fashion. Attention should particularly focus on children who are at or greater than the 95th percentile, and on children who show significant or rapid movement up the growth chart (skipping curves) over time.[22] Electronic medical records often have automatic charting and tracking features for BMI percentile that can aid clinical practice by providing visual cues to initiate conversations about appropriate weight gain with parents and families.[23] Routine well-child care visits are also an excellent time to discuss individual family health behaviors, including family weight history, meal routines, food access, physical activity, sleep habits, and screen time.[24]

Communicating with Parents

Parents are the primary focus for prevention efforts. In infancy and toddler/preschool age groups, results from screening measures should be shared openly with parents, and taking time to develop rapport with the family is important.[25] In early infancy, significant attention is often paid to ensuring adequate weight gain. Parents are concerned if their infant is getting enough to eat and gaining weight. It can difficult to alter the weight gain conversation to a different paradigm focusing on appropriate weight gain. To promote parental self-efficacy to follow recommendations, providers should describe how infancy and the toddler and preschool years are the optimal time to set the stage for lifelong healthy eating habits; this is true for children in all weight categories, but is especially important for families with children who are obese or at risk for becoming obese.

Prevention

Education is the cornerstone of obesity prevention. Providers should deliver concrete suggestions and write them down (or provide preprinted handout materials; **Table 1**) because parents are often trying to absorb a significant amount of information during each well-child visit. Maternal feeding practices are a significant contributor to infant weight gain.[26,27] Helping mothers adhere to established infant feeding guidelines supports appropriate infant feeding and growth. Breastfeeding is recommended for the first year of life and may help reduce the risk of developing overweight and obesity.[28–30] Another important area is a discussion of appropriate food cues. Parents often respond with food when a child cries, rather than using alternative soothing techniques. Given that an infant can become programmed for excessive caloric intake, parents should distinguish cues for hunger (eg, rooting, hand sucking) and resist feeding a child every time the infant cries.[17]

As children grow beyond infancy, key areas for anticipatory education include the timing of introduction of solid foods,[31] resolving picky eating,[31] discussing appropriate portion sizes (see **Table 1**), reviewing recommended amounts of physical activity, healthy sleep habits, and setting appropriate limits on screen time.[18] Each of these factors contributes to the development of obesity. Parents should avoid sugar-sweetened beverages and limit added sugar when possible. Mealtime should not be a battle. By sharing responsibility with the child, parents decide when and what food is presented while children decide whether to eat or how much to eat.[32] Food should not be used as a reward. This practice enhances the value of individual foods for the child and encourages eating in the absence of hunger.[17]

SCHOOL-AGED CHILDREN (AGES 5–12 YEARS)

During the school years, parents continue to influence food intake, sleep, and physical activity. Importantly, ages 5 to 6 years is typically the period of adiposity rebound. Visually reflected on youth growth charts, the adiposity rebound is a (normal) increase in BMI that occurs after BMI has decreased in the first years of life.[33] Early adiposity rebound (before 5.5 years of age) confers a higher risk for adult obesity than later obesity rebound (after 7 years of age).[33]

Screening

School-aged children are considered obese if they are greater than the 95th percentile on CDC growth curves. They are considered overweight if they are more than the 85th percentile for age and sex.[20] Height and weight should be consistently

Table 1
Specific guidance by age group

	Infants/Toddlers/Preschoolers	School Aged	Adolescent	Adult
Portion size	• Guidance on appropriate intake of breast milk or formula • Toddlers and preschoolers need much smaller portions than older children • Refer to www.healthychildren.org for portion size guidance	• Refer to www.healthychildren.org for portion size guidance • Encourage parents to measure portions to ensure correct amounts	• Refer to www.healthychildren.org for portion size guidance • Encourage adolescents to begin attending to portion sizes	• Refer to www.choosemyplate.gov or www.heart.gov • Encourage measurement of portions
Timing of meals/snacks	• Guidance on frequency of feeding and reading infant cues • Toddlers should have 3 meals and up to 2 snacks per day	• 3 meals per day, especially breakfast • Encourage eating when moderately hungry, not when full or overly hungry	• 3 meals per day, especially breakfast • Encourage eating when moderately hungry, not when full or overly hungry	• 3 meals per day, especially breakfast • Encourage eating when moderately hungry, not when full or overly hungry
Nutritional content	• Referral to MyPlate • No juice or sugar-sweetened beverages • Limit added sugars	• Referral to MyPlate • No juice or sugar-sweetened beverages • Limit added sugars	• Referral to MyPlate • No juice or sugar-sweetened beverages • Limit added sugars	• Referral to MyPlate • No juice or sugar-sweetened beverages • Limit added sugars
Introduction of new foods	• No introduction of solid foods until 6 mo of age • Guidance on development of picky eating in toddlers and information on importance of tasting (even without swallowing) a new food 10–15 times before acceptance	• Guidance on picky eating and information on importance of tasting (even without swallowing) a new food 10–15 times before acceptance • Introduce a variety of foods and flavors • Involve children in meal planning, shopping, and meal preparation	• Encourage a wide variety of foods, especially fruits and vegetables • Involve adolescents in meal planning, shopping, and meal preparation	• Continue introducing new foods for a varied and healthful diet

(continued on next page)

	Infants/Toddlers/ Preschoolers	School Aged	Adolescent	Adult
Table 1 *(continued)*				
Physical activity	• Toddler: 90 min/d • Preschool: 120 min/d	• ≥60 min/d	• 150 min/wk	• 150 min/wk
Sleep	• Infants: 12–14 h/d including regular naps • Toddlers: 12 h/d including at least 1 nap • Preschoolers: 11 h/d	• 10–11 h of quality sleep per night	• 9–10 h of quality sleep per night	• 7–8 h of quality sleep per night
Screen time	• None before 2 y • >age 2 y, max 2 h/d	• Maximum 2 h/d	• Maximum 2 h/d	• Maximum 2 h/d
Motivational interviewing	• What are some of your hopes for your child's health now and as he/she grows up? • How do you think your family's approach to eating and physical activity supports those goals?		• If you could wave a magic wand and achieve your top 2 goals, what would those be? If you woke up tomorrow and those things were accomplished, how would your life be different? • How do your health and the way you care for your body affect those goals?	

measured and recorded at every physician visit to allow for accurate tracking over time and to help to identify children who are at risk for the development of obesity. BMI percentile as the sole indicator of obesity and obesity risk has limitations. BMI percentile does not distinguish well between adiposity and muscularity.[34] Other indicators of central adiposity (eg, waist/height ratio[34]) and health (eg, insulin resistance, blood pressure, and lipid profile) help to identify children with metabolic syndrome who would benefit from aggressive lifestyle interventions.[18] Additional screening questions include family weight history, and family and child health habits. School-aged children should be screened for mood and behavior problems with a tool such as such as the Pediatric Symptoms Checklist[35] because affective disorders often accompany obesity.

Communication

Communication between caregivers, children, and their families requires care and empathy while using appropriate language and nonverbal communication. It is important to focus on health and healthy behaviors rather than solely on the child's weight. Terms such as healthy weight, at risk for overweight, or overweight are less pejorative and help facilitate conversation.[24] Providers should also assess the family's readiness to change and their willingness to receive information. Using motivational interviewing techniques, simple inquiries about where they think they are doing well, and where they would like to improve can help establish shared goals for eating, physical activity, sleep, and screen time (see **Table 1**). School-aged children understand such conversations and should be included. Frame the discussion in terms of health behaviors rather than weight. Identify 1 or 2 important target behaviors rather than suggesting that the family make wholesale behavioral changes.[24]

Prevention

Providing sensitive feedback on the child's weight status and risk, as well as appropriate education on the importance of establishing healthy behaviors and routines, is a key part of prevention in school-aged children. When possible, parents should identify and set achievable goals within the context of their individual family situation (see **Table 1**). Written goals are more likely to translate into concrete behavioral changes. Identifying likely barriers also helps sustain adherence to recommended behavioral change. Key areas of prevention include minimizing (or eliminating) sugar-sweetened beverage use, limiting screen time, ensuring a regular meal schedule including breakfast, ensuring sufficient sleep, and increasing physical activity.

ADOLESCENTS (AGES 13–18 YEARS)

Adolescence, around the time of puberty, is a risk period for excessive weight gain. The hormonal and physical changes of puberty often lead to changes in body composition[36] and eating behaviors.[37] These changes also heighten genetic risk for disordered eating.[38] Adolescence is a time when youth are developing autonomy from their parents.[39] This autonomy likely includes more independence in food choices and ad libitum consumption. Adolescents have lower abilities to self-regulate caloric intake compared with adults.[40] Alterations in brain neurochemistry during adolescence affect executive functioning. Encouragingly, adolescence represents a sensitive period during which alterations in white and gray matter are susceptible to intervention.[40] Adolescence therefore is a high-risk, high-reward period of development in the context of obesity prevention.

Screening

Overweight adolescents are between the 85th and 95th BMI percentiles for age and sex. Obese adolescents are greater than or equal to the 95th percentile. Severely obese adolescents are greater than or equal to the 120th percentile.[41] Screening for metabolic syndrome and using other indicators metabolic risk (such as waist/height ratio) helps classify risk and target potential interventions. It is important to assess family history and family health environment for adolescent patients. It is also important to assess the individual health habits of adolescent patients because they tend to spend more time away from home to engage in eating and physical activity behaviors.[31] Adolescents' sleep habits are often suboptimal,[42] and a conversation about normal sleep habits is important. Mental health comorbidities are more common in overweight or obese adolescents. Screen for mood disorders, anxiety, and attention disorders during routine office visits and refer to behavioral specialists as needed.

Communication

Communication with adolescent patients can be particularly challenging. Physical appearance, difference from others, and sensitivity to teasing are common in this age group.[43] Framing all discussion in terms of health behaviors is important. Avoid using pejorative terms, such as fat or skinny. Avoid lecturing or making patients defensive. Engage adolescents in a conversation about realistic goals and their desire to change. Assessing an individual adolescent's readiness to change is as critical as assessing parent and family readiness to change.

Prevention

The targets for prevention (see **Table 1**) are the same for adolescents as for younger children. However, conversations about addressing motivation and willingness to change take on even more importance. Brief motivational interviewing strategies can help elicit willingness to change and identify primary behavioral targets (see **Table 1**). Adolescents are often technologically literate and may find apps and m-health tools appealing. Fitness trackers (eg, Fitbit, Jawbone UP) or apps for tracking food intake (eg, My Fitness Pal, Lose It) have more appeal in this age group. Although prevention strategies for adolescents should focus on the individual, engaging the family is important to ensure that changes made are family-wide and encouraged by other members of the family.

ADULTS

Although obesity is often an established health condition for adults, there are several at-risk time periods for developing obesity. In particular, the perinatal period,[44,45] the initiation of some psychiatric medications, traumatic life events, or the onset of depression with associated development of maladaptive eating behaviors[46] are periods in which individuals are at particular risk for developing obesity as adults.

Screening

BMI is the primary indicator of overweight and obesity in adulthood. Individuals with a BMI of greater than or equal to 25 are considered overweight. Individuals with a BMI greater than or equal to 30 are obese, and individuals with a BMI greater than or equal to 40 are severely (morbidly) obese. Waist circumference, neck circumference, and other indicators of metabolic syndrome are helpful baseline screening elements. Actuarial tables providing weight ranges for height are another way to conceptualize a healthy weight range depending on an individual's gender, height, and body frame.

Communication

A nonjudgmental approach to discussing weight using neutral language, evaluating motivation and readiness for change, and a focus on future behaviors rather than past missteps is critical.[25,47] Although this is a sensitive topic, providers should not avoid discussing weight and associated health consequences of excess weight for overweight or obese patients.[47] Motivational interviewing remains a particularly useful technique for communicating with adult patients and enhancing motivation for change (see **Table 1**).[48,49]

Prevention

Table 1 provides a summary of recommendations for preventive behaviors in adults. As with younger populations, family and social support is important.[50] Assessing and promoting social support and encouraging adults to work with significant others to improve health behaviors enhances preventive efforts. Electronic tools are also helpful for adults trying to improve health behaviors. Self-monitoring is a powerful tool for weight management and several tracking apps exist to monitor nutritional intake (eg, My Fitness Pal, Lose It), physical activity (eg, Run Keeper, Fitbit, Jawbone UP), and sleep (eg, Fitbit, Jawbone UP, SleepBot).

SPECIAL POPULATIONS: AUTISTIC SPECTRUM DISORDER AND MILD TRAUMATIC BRAIN INJURY

The pediatric special needs population, including children with autistic spectrum disorder (ASD), is especially prone to obesity[51,52] because of a tendency to inactivity and difficulty with participating in structured physical activities,[53] rigid preferences for certain foods and textures,[54] and medication effects.[55] There seems to be a particular propensity for obesity in children with ASD,[56] among whom up to 25% of children are overweight or obese.[51] Among behaviorally challenged children with ASD, atypical antipsychotic medications are often used[57] with the untoward effect of an associated increase in weight, likely driven by an increase in appetite.[55,58] Anticipatory guidance for parents of children with ASD can help minimize undue weight gain and the associated metabolic consequences. Behavioral programs designed for obese children without special needs have been successfully applied to children with ASD and intellectual disabilities.[59] Without appropriate intervention, patients with ASD have higher rates of obesity and the associated comorbidities.[60]

Other populations, such as patients with mild traumatic brain injury (or concussion), are prone to deconditioning caused by inactivity.[61] More than 3 million concussions are reported each year.[62] Traditional management recommends physical and cognitive rest to enhance recovery and minimize risk of recurrence.[63] Fears of the possible long-term neurologic effects from concussions have led some parents to remove their children from sports and activities.[64] However, evidence to date has not shown that withdrawal from sports or physical or cognitively challenging activities is brain protective. It has also not been shown to shorten concussion recovery times or improve outcomes. Early reengagement and activity after minor head injury seems to aid in recovery.[65,66] In addition, there is no evidence that single or multiple youth sports–related concussion consistently leads to any long-term neurocognitive challenges. Youth sports involvement, including youth football, is extremely safe. Central nervous system–related death in youth sports is less likely than repeated lightning strikes.[67] Youth sports provide a foundation of healthy play and teamwork, and the benefits are well established.[68] In addition, exercise benefits the developing brain with attributable benefits in attention, memory, and mood.[69]

Primary care providers should counsel families of special needs populations regarding the safety and benefits of exercise and the importance of healthy nutrition. Unless other reasons for avoiding physical activity are identified (eg, cardiovascular risk factors such as medication exposure and long QT syndrome, or atlantoaxial instability), individuals should be encouraged to exercise. Doing so promotes long-term physical fitness, and prevents the onset of obesity-related disease.

CULTURAL CONSIDERATIONS

The percentage and distribution of adiposity for a given BMI varies by race and ethnicity.[70] BMI therefore should not be used as a universal proxy for adiposity. Screens for obesity should include additional measures, such as body fat percentage, waist circumference, and indicators of the metabolic syndrome. In addition, behavioral screening tools should be culturally appropriate when assessing mood, body image, and eating behaviors in diverse groups.[71] If culturally specific measurements are not available, providers should use language that is culturally sensitive and specific.

Another important point for consideration is that perspectives regarding shape and weight vary among different cultural groups. This variation may create barriers to conversation and engaging in behavioral change. Parents of children from various racial/ethnic groups may not view their children as overweight or obese by accepted medical standards. As an example, Latina mothers are less likely to report their children as being overweight or obese, even if they meet established BMI criteria.[72,73] In addition, in the absence of tangible medical complications, some individuals might have limited motivation to address weight-related concerns.[74,75] Racial and ethnic minorities are not homogenous. Significant within-group differences also exist. These considerations should be taken into account when establishing rapport engaging in any health-related conversation.

SUMMARY

Obesity prevention across the lifespan is vital. Each developmental period provides unique challenges and opportunities to improve health. Primary care providers have a critical role in screening, conveying important information to families, and providing tools for prevention. This relationship between provider and patient should be based on trust and have good lines of culturally appropriate communication. There are many resources available for patients and families who are trying to improve their health online, and through mobile applications. Other important resources include families, communities, and health care providers. Behavioral change is difficult and takes time. However, a good working relationship between patient and provider, tailored information to individuals, and addressing motivational issues have the potential to greatly reduce the incidence of obesity and improve the health of our nation.

REFERENCES

1. Tsai AG, Williamson DF, Glick HA. Direct medical cost of overweight and obesity in the USA: a quantitative systematic review. Obes Rev 2011;12(1):50–61.
2. Clinical guidelines on the identification, evaluation, and treatment of overweight and obesity in adults–the evidence report. National Institutes of Health. Obes Res 1998;6(Suppl 2):51S–209S.
3. Pulgaron ER. Childhood obesity: a review of increased risk for physical and psychological comorbidities. Clin Ther 2013;35(1):A18–32.
4. Schwimmer JB, Burwinkle TM, Varni JW. Health-related quality of life of severely obese children and adolescents. JAMA 2003;289(14):1813–9.
5. Ebbeling CB, Pawlak DB, Ludwig DS. Childhood obesity: public-health crisis, common sense cure. Lancet 2002;360(9331):473–82.
6. Must A, Jacques PF, Dallal GE, et al. Long-term morbidity and mortality of overweight adolescents. A follow-up of the Harvard Growth Study of 1922 to 1935. N Engl J Med 1992;327(19):1350–5.
7. Wijga AH, Scholtens S, Bemelmans WJ, et al. Comorbidities of obesity in school children: a cross-sectional study in the PIAMA birth cohort. BMC Public Health 2010;10:184.
8. Finkelstein EA, Khavjou OA, Thompson H, et al. Obesity and severe obesity forecasts through 2030. Am J Prev Med 2012;42(6):563–70.
9. Finkelstein EA, Trogdon JG, Cohen JW, et al. Annual medical spending attributable to obesity: payer-and service-specific estimates. Health Aff (Millwood) 2009;28(5):w822–31.
10. Oude Luttikhuis H, Baur L, Jansen H, et al. Interventions for treating obesity in children. Cochrane Database Syst Rev 2009;(1):CD001872.
11. Ells LJ, Campbell K, Lidstone J, et al. Prevention of childhood obesity. Best Pract Res Clin Endocrinol Metab 2005;19(3):441–54.
12. Lobstein T, Baur L, Uauy R. Obesity in children and young people: a crisis in public health. Obes Rev 2004;5(Suppl 1):4–104.

13. Birch LL, Anzman-Frasca S, Paul IM. Starting early: obesity prevention during infancy. Nestle Nutr Inst Workshop Ser 2012;73:81–94.

14. Ong KK, Ahmed ML, Emmett PM, et al. Association between postnatal catch-up growth and obesity in childhood: prospective cohort study. BMJ 2000;320(7240): 967–71.

15. Stettler N, Zemel BS, Kumanyika S, et al. Infant weight gain and childhood overweight status in a multicenter, cohort study. Pediatrics 2002;109(2):194–9.

16. Taveras EM, Rifas-Shiman SL, Belfort MB, et al. Weight status in the first 6 months of life and obesity at 3 years of age. Pediatrics 2009;123(4):1177–83.

17. Paul IM, Savage JS, Anzman SL, et al. Preventing obesity during infancy: a pilot study. Obesity (Silver Spring) 2011;19(2):353–61.

18. Rome ES. Obesity prevention and treatment. Pediatr Rev 2011;32(9):363–72.

19. de Onis M, Onyango AW, Borghi E, et al. Development of a WHO growth reference for school-aged children and adolescents. Bull World Health Organ 2007; 85(9):660–7.

20. CDC. Clinical growth charts. 2009. Available at: http://www.cdc.gov/growthcharts/clinical_charts.htm. Accessed May 19, 2015.

21. Peirson L, Fitzpatrick-Lewis D, Morrison K, et al. Treatment of overweight and obesity in children and youth: a systematic review and meta-analysis. CMAJ Open 2015;3(1):E35–46.

22. McGuire S. Institute of Medicine. 2013. Evaluating obesity prevention efforts: a plan for measuring progress. Washington, DC: The National Academies Press, 2013. Adv Nutr 2014;5(2):191–2.

23. Flower KB, Perrin EM, Viadro CI, et al. Using body mass index to identify overweight children: barriers and facilitators in primary care. Ambul Pediatr 2007; 7(1):38–44.

24. Perrin EM, Finkle JP, Benjamin JT. Obesity prevention and the primary care pediatrician's office. Curr Opin Pediatr 2007;19(3):354–61.

25. Farnesi BC, Ball GD, Newton AS. Family-health professional relations in pediatric weight management: an integrative review. Pediatr Obes 2012;7(3):175–86.

26. Rodgers RF, Paxton SJ, Massey R, et al. Maternal feeding practices predict weight gain and obesogenic eating behaviors in young children: a prospective study. Int J Behav Nutr Phys Act 2013;10:24.

27. Worobey J, Lopez MI, Hoffman DJ. Maternal behavior and infant weight gain in the first year. J Nutr Educ Behav 2009;41(3):169–75.

28. Beyerlein A, von Kries R. Breastfeeding and body composition in children: will there ever be conclusive empirical evidence for a protective effect against overweight? Am J Clin Nutr 2011;94(6 Suppl):1772S–5S.

29. Hansstein FV. The impact of breastfeeding on early childhood obesity: evidence from the national survey of children's health. Am J Health Promot 2015. [Epub ahead of print].

30. Section on Breastfeeding. Breastfeeding and the use of human milk. Pediatrics 2012;129(3):e827–41.

31. Webber L, Hill C, Saxton J, et al. Eating behaviour and weight in children. Int J Obes (Lond) 2009;33(1):21–8.

32. Satter E. Ellyn Satter's division of responsibility in feeding. 2015. Available at: http://ellynsatterinstitute.org/cms-assets/documents/203702-180136.dor-2015-2.pdf. Accessed May 27, 2015.

33. Rolland-Cachera MF, Deheeger M, Bellisle F, et al. Adiposity rebound in children: a simple indicator for predicting obesity. Am J Clin Nutr 1984;39(1): 129–35.

34. Ashwell M, Hsieh SD. Six reasons why the waist-to-height ratio is a rapid and effective global indicator for health risks of obesity and how its use could simplify the international public health message on obesity. Int J Food Sci Nutr 2005; 56(5):303–7.
35. Jellinek MS, Murphy JM, Robinson J, et al. Pediatric Symptom Checklist: screening school-age children for psychosocial dysfunction. J Pediatr 1988; 112(2):201–9.
36. Mihalopoulos NL, Holubkov R, Young P, et al. Expected changes in clinical measures of adiposity during puberty. J Adolesc Health 2010;47(4):360–6.
37. Shomaker LB, Tanofsky-Kraff M, Savastano DM, et al. Puberty and observed energy intake: boy, can they eat! Am J Clin Nutr 2010;92(1):123–9.
38. Klump KL, Keel PK, Sisk C, et al. Preliminary evidence that estradiol moderates genetic influences on disordered eating attitudes and behaviors during puberty. Psychol Med 2010;40(10):1745–53.
39. Steinberg L, Silverberg SB. The vicissitudes of autonomy in early adolescence. Child Dev 1986;57(4):841–51.
40. Johnson SL, Taylor-Holloway LA. Non-Hispanic white and Hispanic elementary school children's self-regulation of energy intake. Am J Clin Nutr 2006;83(6): 1276–82.
41. Maring B, Greenspan LC, Chandra M, et al. Comparing US paediatric and adult weight classification at the transition from late teenage to young adulthood. Pediatr Obes 2015;10:371–9.
42. National Heart Lung and Blood Institute. Research NCoSD. Problem sleepiness in your patient. Bethesda (MD): National Institutes of Health; 1997. Available at: www.nhlbi.nih.gov/files/docs/resources/sleep/pslp_pat.pdf.
43. Libbey HP, Story MT, Neumark-Sztainer DR, et al. Teasing, disordered eating behaviors, and psychological morbidities among overweight adolescents. Obesity (Silver Spring) 2008;16(Suppl 2):S24–9.
44. Gunderson EP, Abrams B, Selvin S. The relative importance of gestational gain and maternal characteristics associated with the risk of becoming overweight after pregnancy. Int J Obes Relat Metab Disord 2000;24(12):1660–8.
45. Mamun AA, Kinarivala M, O'Callaghan MJ, et al. Associations of excess weight gain during pregnancy with long-term maternal overweight and obesity: evidence from 21 y postpartum follow-up. Am J Clin Nutr 2010;91(5):1336–41.
46. Faubel M. Body image and depression in women with early and late onset obesity. J Psychol 1989;123(4):385–95.
47. Lyznicki JM, Young DC, Riggs JA, et al. Obesity: assessment and management in primary care. Am Fam Physician 2001;63(11):2185–96.
48. Artinian NT, Fletcher GF, Mozaffarian D, et al. Interventions to promote physical activity and dietary lifestyle changes for cardiovascular risk factor reduction in adults: a scientific statement from the American Heart Association. Circulation 2010;122(4):406–41.
49. West DS, DiLillo V, Bursac Z, et al. Motivational interviewing improves weight loss in women with type 2 diabetes. Diabetes Care 2007;30(5):1081–7.
50. Puhl RM, Brownell KD. Confronting and coping with weight stigma: an investigation of overweight and obese adults. Obesity (Silver Spring) 2006;14(10):1802–15.
51. Broder-Fingert S, Brazauskas K, Lindgren K, et al. Prevalence of overweight and obesity in a large clinical sample of children with autism. Acad Pediatr 2014; 14(4):408–14.
52. Chen AY, Kim SE, Houtrow AJ, et al. Prevalence of obesity among children with chronic conditions. Obesity (Silver Spring) 2010;18(1):210–3.

53. Pan CY. Objectively measured physical activity between children with autism spectrum disorders and children without disabilities during inclusive recess settings in Taiwan. J Autism Dev Disord 2008;38(7):1292–301.

54. Schreck KA, Williams K, Smith AF. A comparison of eating behaviors between children with and without autism. J Autism Dev Disord 2004;34(4):433–8.

55. McCracken JT, McGough J, Shah B, et al. Risperidone in children with autism and serious behavioral problems. N Engl J Med 2002;347(5):314–21.

56. Egan AM, Dreyer ML, Odar CC, et al. Obesity in young children with autism spectrum disorders: prevalence and associated factors. Child Obes 2013;9(2):125–31.

57. Mandell DS, Morales KH, Marcus SC, et al. Psychotropic medication use among Medicaid-enrolled children with autism spectrum disorders. Pediatrics 2008; 121(3):e441–8.

58. Politte LC, McDougle CJ. Atypical antipsychotics in the treatment of children and adolescents with pervasive developmental disorders. Psychopharmacology 2014;231(6):1023–36.

59. Hinckson EA, Dickinson A, Water T, et al. Physical activity, dietary habits and overall health in overweight and obese children and youth with intellectual disability or autism. Res Dev Disabil 2013;34(4):1170–8.

60. Croen LA, Zerbo O, Qian Y, et al. The health status of adults on the autism spectrum. Autism 2015. [Epub ahead of print].

61. Silverberg ND, Iverson GL. Is rest after concussion "the best medicine?": recommendations for activity resumption following concussion in athletes, civilians, and military service members. J Head Trauma Rehabil 2013;28(4):250–9.

62. Khurana VG, Kaye AH. An overview of concussion in sport. J Clin Neurosci 2012; 19(1):1–11.

63. DeMatteo C, Stazyk K, Singh SK, et al. Development of a conservative protocol to return children and youth to activity following concussive injury. Clin Pediatr 2015; 54(2):152–63.

64. Fainaru S, Fainaru-Wada M. Youth football participation drops. Outside the lines 2013. Available at: http://espn.go.com/espn/otl/story/_/page/popwarner/pop-warner-youth-football-participation-drops-nfl-concussion-crisis-seen-causal-factor. Accessed June 15, 2015.

65. McCrea M, Guskiewicz K, Randolph C, et al. Effects of a symptom-free waiting period on clinical outcome and risk of reinjury after sport-related concussion. Neurosurgery 2009;65(5):876–82 [discussion: 882–3].

66. Thomas DG, Apps JN, Hoffmann RG, et al. Benefits of strict rest after acute concussion: a randomized controlled trial. Pediatrics 2015;135(2):213–23.

67. Kirkwood MW, Randolph C, Yeates KO. Sport-related concussion: a call for evidence and perspective amidst the alarms. Clin J Sport Med 2012;22(5):383–4.

68. Smith JJ, Eather N, Morgan PJ, et al. The health benefits of muscular fitness for children and adolescents: a systematic review and meta-analysis. Sports Med 2014;44(9):1209–23.

69. Cerillo-Urbina AJ, Garcia-Hermoso A, Sanchez-Lopez M, et al. The effects of physical exercise in children with attention deficit hyperactivity disorder: a systematic review and meta-analysis of randomized control trials. Child Care Health Dev 2015. [Epub ahead of print].

70. Rahman M, Temple JR, Breitkopf CR, et al. Racial differences in body fat distribution among reproductive-aged women. Metabolism 2009;58(9):1329–37.

71. Cassidy O, Sbrocco T, Tanofsky-Kraff M. Utilizing non-traditional research designs to explore culture-specific risk factors for eating disorders in African American adolescents. Adv Eat Disord 2015;3(1):91–102.

72. Hackie M, Bowles CL. Maternal perception of their overweight children. Public Health Nurs 2007;24(6):538–46.
73. Lindsay AC, Sussner KM, Greaney ML, et al. Latina mothers' beliefs and practices related to weight status, feeding, and the development of child overweight. Public Health Nurs 2011;28(2):107–18.
74. Burnet DL, Plaut AJ, Ossowski K, et al. Community and family perspectives on addressing overweight in urban, African-American youth. J Gen Intern Med 2008;23(2):175–9.
75. Sbrocco T, Carter MM, Lewis EL, et al. Church-based obesity treatment for African-American women improves adherence. Ethn Dis 2005;15(2):246–55.

Multidisciplinary Teams and Obesity

Role of the Modern Patient-Centered Medical Home

Kevin M. Bernstein, MD, MMS[a,b], Debra A. Manning, MD, MBA[c,d,*],
Regina M. Julian, MHA, MBA[e]

KEYWORDS

- Obesity management • Primary care • Patient-centered medical home

KEY POINTS

- Interdisciplinary teams within patient-centered medical homes (PCMH) can effectively screen for obesity and provide sustainable treatment options with close follow-up to achieve greater weight loss.
- Behavioral health plays a major role in effective weight loss. Embedded behavioral health specialists in PCMH teams offer an expanded variety of behavioral modifications.
- Behaviorally based treatments are safe and effective for weight loss and maintenance.

INTRODUCTION

The concept of the modern patient-centered medical home (PCMH) began in 1967 when the American Academy of Pediatrics used the term "medical home" to describe the role of primary care pediatricians in the treatment of children with chronic

Disclosure Statement: The authors have nothing to disclose.
The views expressed in this article are those of the author and do not necessarily reflect the official policy or position of the Department of the Navy, Department of Defense, nor the US Government.
We are employees of the US Government. This work was prepared as part of our official duties. Title 17, USC, §105 provides that 'Copyright protection under this title is not available for any work of the US Government.' Title 17, USC, §101 defines a US Government work as a work prepared by a military service member or employee of the US Government as part of that person's official duties.
^a Medical Corps, United States Navy, PSC 482, Box 2569, FPO, AP 96362-2500, USA; ^b Fleet Surgical Team SEVEN, Okinawa, Japan; ^c Medical Corps, United States Navy; ^d Medical Home Port, Bureau of Medicine and Surgery, 7700 Arlington Boulevard, Falls Church, VA 22042, USA; ^e Primary Care (Patient Centered Medical Home), Clinical Support Division, Defense Health Agency, 7700 Arlington Boulevard, Falls Church, VA 22042, USA
* Corresponding author. Medical Home Port, Bureau of Medicine and Surgery, 7700 Arlington Boulevard, Falls Church, VA 22042.
E-mail address: dr.deb.manning@gmail.com

Prim Care Clin Office Pract 43 (2016) 53–59
http://dx.doi.org/10.1016/j.pop.2015.08.010
0095-4543/16/$ – see front matter Published by Elsevier Inc.

conditions.[1] Over time, the medical home has evolved into a model of health care delivery applicable to all—not just children or those with chronic conditions. The PCMH consists of 7 core principles: a personal physician, team-based care led by a primary care physician, a whole-person orientation, care that is coordinated across the health care system, enhanced quality and safety through the use and integration of new technology, enhanced access to care, and new payment methods to reflect care that is value added.[2]

With American health care in a period of massive transition, the PCMH model has transformed both small practices and large health care systems. The PCMH model has also become an attractive mechanism to deliver quality health care at a lower cost. Several studies show that PCMH teams effectively provide high-quality care with increased patient satisfaction and reduced costs.[3–8] The PCMH model has been correspondingly endorsed by multiple medical societies including the American Academy of Pediatrics, American Academy of Family Physicians, American College of Physicians, and the American Osteopathic Association.[2]

One in 3 American adults are obese (defined as a body mass index of >30 kg/m^2).[9] The prevalence of obesity has increased by more than 130% since the late 1970s[10] and continues to rise. Addressing the chronic public health challenges posed by increasing rates of obesity is a priority for primary care physicians working within interdisciplinary teams. Obesity leads to increases in mortality, coronary artery disease, type 2 diabetes mellitus, certain cancers, musculoskeletal injuries/chronic pain, maternal and fetal complications during pregnancy, and other diseases.[11]

The US Preventive Services Task Force recommends primary care clinicians offer obese adult interventions to help promote weight loss.[11] With practices transforming to PCMH models across the United States, teams are well-positioned to provide necessary services to combat preventable comorbidities associated with obesity as well.

It is difficult for most primary care physicians to dedicate sufficient time and resources to accomplish meaningful behavioral changes for patients desiring to lose weight or reduce the risk of chronic disease purely on their own.[12] A team of health care professionals from multiple disciplines can provide more comprehensive value and evidence-based care that is proven to combat obesity and other preventable diseases. Structured behavioral counseling for weight loss can be provided by a variety of trained specialists in the PCMH setting.[13,14]

The Patient-Centered Medical Home Model: A Personal Physician for Everyone

A specific primary care physician should lead the PCMH health care team and help to structure individualized plans for patient care.[14] A thorough personal, family, occupational, and social history should include a review of current medications known to cause weight gain, use of over-the-counter herbal or sports supplements, a behavioral health history, and physical activity patterns.[14] An appropriate physical examination with indicated ancillary testing can rule out organic causes of obesity (eg, thyroid disease). In the context of team-based care, primary care physicians are best suited to manage complex comorbidities such as diabetes, hypertension, hyperlipidemia, cardiovascular disease, depression, and anxiety.[14,15] Primary care physicians are also best positioned to initiate conversations about the decision to pursue adjunctive medication therapy[12] or to initiate bariatric surgical consultation.[15] Working with the rest of the PCMH team, primary care physicians are then best able to construct and coordinate safe courses of action to meet the needs of each patient for an individualized and comprehensive weight loss plan.[15]

The Patient-Centered Medical Home: The Important Role of Behavioral Health

Behavioral health plays a foundational role in initiating and sustaining effective weight loss.[13] Although primary care physicians typically have the training necessary to provide behavioral therapy,[12] time constraints often necessitate referral to behavioral therapy specialists for more comprehensive and intensive behavioral interventions.[12]

Behavioral health specialists (psychologists, social workers, psychiatrists) offer a breadth of services to help patients identify barriers to change and modify existing behaviors to achieve agreed upon weight loss goals.[12,13,15] Behavioral specialists can also help patients to identify specific self-monitoring mechanisms and strategies for to maintain a target weight once a specific goal is achieved.[12] Embedding behavioral health within the PCMH, enhances care coordination and increases the likelihood of meaningful patient-centered behavioral change.[14]

The Patient-Centered Medical Home: Where Does Nutrition Fit in?

Setting realistic goals and providing mechanisms for tracking daily caloric intake that are not overbearing and fit within the patient's lifestyle helps to promote the caloric deficit necessary to achieve meaningful weight loss.[12] Registered dietitians, in particular, play a significant role in helping to shape dietary recommendations using an individualized, patient-centered approach.[15]

Behavioral health impacts nutritional support as well, because patients often turn to food as a coping mechanism for different life stressors.[12] Behavioral interventions help patients to stay motivated and make healthy choices when dealing with stress.

Coordinated nutritional support is especially important for patients who have specific dietary needs based on specific medical conditions (eg, celiac disease, food allergies, food intolerances, diabetes mellitus, vitamin deficiencies, and anemia). Patients who have undergone bariatric surgery or colonic resection also benefit from the involvement of a nutrition professional. Age and gender (eg, folate for women of childbearing age and calcium/vitamin D supplementation in older patients), and medication side effects (eg, green leafy vegetables and warfarin) are other factors that must be considered in a comprehensive obesity management program.[15]

Physical Activity: Help from the Medical Home?

Physical therapists, occupational therapists, exercise physiologists, personal trainers, and other professionals are available to help patients establish safe and effective plans to promote and sustain healthy levels of physical activity.[12] Rather than providing a one-size-fits all approach to physical activity (eg, 150 minutes per week of moderate-intensity exercise), a patient-centered approach is preferred. This strategy is especially true for patients with chronic pain, current musculoskeletal injury, cardiac and/or pulmonary disease, or any other condition impacting their ability to exercise.[15] Specific activities can be safely tailored to patient preference to enhance adherence and promote weight loss.[15]

OTHER PLAYERS ON THE PATIENT-CENTERED MEDICAL HOME TEAM

Other members of the PCMH team can play critical roles to support patients in their weight management efforts. Case managers can help to identify and overcome specific social barriers. Other behavioral health providers can help to overcome mental or emotional barriers associated with lifestyle modifications.[12,13,15] Primary care physicians help to quarterback the team. Physician guidance also helps to determine appropriate levels of physical activity, particularly for cardiac rehabilitation patients.[13]

Pharmacologic Monitoring Within the Patient-Centered Medical Home

Many transformed practices embed pharmacists within the PCMH team to help monitor medication use, interactions, side effects, and therapeutic benefit. Patients who make positive lifestyle changes often have altered requirements for certain medications. Dosages need to be adjusted or drugs may become unnecessary as metabolic profiles improve. For example, an obese patient on multiple antihypertensive medications starts a personalized, multidisciplinary treatment plan. Alterations in physical activity and diet lead to weight loss and metabolic improvements. Monitoring blood pressure and adjusting medication dosing is something that can be safely done by the team pharmacist.[13] An embedded pharmacist can make recommendations for dosage adjustments, elimination of certain medications, and also help to track metabolic parameters.

Case Management in the Patient-Centered Medical Home Setting

Case management helps patients to incorporate lifestyle modifications by coordinating community services and interdisciplinary care. As an example, case managers can help patients to find child care or vocational services and financial resources. There may be cases where a patient may live in a rural community with limited resources.[16] In some cases, they may live in an unsafe neighborhood. A case manager may be able to help identify safe places for patients to exercise. They may help to identify different organizations such as running clubs, support groups, or sports clubs to engage in social aspects of community-based physical activity.

Asynchronous Communication: Patient Centered to Keep Everyone in the Loop

Expanding technologies provide an array of options for provider–patient communications. Secure messaging allows for direct communication between patients and the PCMH team.[17] Mobile applications monitor activity, diet, and other metrics to give patients real-time feedback based on individual goals.[18,19] Telemedicine and video conferencing are other options for provider–patient communications to help patients initiate and sustain behavioral change and necessary lifestyle modifications.[16,20,21]

Group Visits

Gathering patients with similar interests provides a support network that extends beyond the practice and into the community. Meeting with groups of patients who have similar disease states (eg, diabetes, hyperlipidemia, obesity) is an efficient way for the PCMH team to deliver a unified message within an open forum where patients can share experiences and questions. Patients wishing to lose weight are more likely to be successful if they meet regularly with peers and with their team.[12] Group visits are another mechanism to provide ongoing support to help patients meet their stated goals.

CLINICAL CORRELATION

In 2011, the Centers for Medicare and Medicaid Services approved reimbursement for primary care physicians to provide intensive behavioral health counseling.[15] Counseling can be provided over the course of 6 months for obese patients in primary care settings, covering 14 in-person sessions lasting 10 to 15 minutes each.[22] Lifestyle "coaches" have also been used to help treat patients with obesity.[23] One study used medical assistants trained to provide 8 coaching sessions over the course of 6 months. The control group lost 0.9 kg and the intervention group lost 4.4 kg.[23] In another randomized trial of 390 obese adults in 6 primary care practices. One-third of the patients receiving enhanced lifestyle coaching achieved meaningful weight loss. This program featured quarterly visits with the individual's primary care physician, monthly visits to a lifestyle coach combined with either orlistat, sibutramine, or meal replacements.[24] A systematic review of 58 trials found that behaviorally based treatment resulted in 3 kg (6.6 lb) more weight loss compared with controls after 12 to 18 months.[11] Participation in more treatment sessions was associated with greater weight loss. One of the limitations in most prior studies is that few report health outcomes and few were conducted in traditional primary care offices. Additionally, follow-up after 18 months is lacking and none of the studies included individuals with a mean body mass index of greater than 40 kg/m^2.

A recent systematic review of 12 trials involving 3893 participants found that patients who received medication, increased physical activity, and engaged in behavioral therapy achieved greater weight loss than patients engaged in programs lacking one or more of these individual components.[22] Patients who attended more sessions (telephone and in person) lost more weight and were more likely to lose 5% or more of their baseline weight. Interdisciplinary collaboration with a variety of trained professionals (eg, behavioral therapy, nutrition) was provided by telephone or in person. Collaborative sessions were effective and sustainable for obese patients seen in the primary care setting.

SUMMARY/DISCUSSION

The US Preventive Services Task Force recommends that clinicians should screen adults for obesity. Consider referring patients with a body mass index of 30 kg/m^2 or higher to intensive, multicomponent behavioral interventions (grade B recommendation).[12] Referral to specialized academic medical centers is another option for ongoing intensive treatment.[25] A comprehensive, interdisciplinary team includes multiple health care professionals including behavioral health providers, registered dietitians, exercise physiologists, and other allied health care personnel.[25]

Outside of academic centers, longitudinal multidisciplinary care can be accomplished in the context of the modern PCMH staffed with professionals to support such care under 1 roof.[14] Using the PCMH model, primary care physicians may be able to provide direct services to patients using a local fitness center or gym. This model potentially represents a form of direct primary care payment plan.[26,27] Many fitness centers, gyms, and rehabilitation centers have on-site health care professionals already (multi-D reference). Some orthopedic centers have physician-owned physical and occupational therapy on site for treatment and postoperative rehabilitation.[28] A similar PCMH model would provide all support services for lifestyle modifications in one building.

Although guidelines continue to recommend face-to-face encounters for counseling sessions, telephone or social media follow-up may be just as effective,[16,20,21] at a lower cost and greater convenience for the PCMH team and the patient.[16] Technology-based interventions can also increase access and decrease costs of care for patients in underserved communities.[16] Secure electronic messaging,[17,19] smart phone devices, and mobile applications[18] are asynchronous forms of communication that can be used to provide ongoing motivation and continuity of care.

Coordination of care by the PCMH team potentially decreases fragmentation of care, increases convenience for the patient, and decreases unnecessary costs. Multidisciplinary collaboration between primary care physicians and other trained health professionals within PCMH represents an attractive approach for the sustainable treatment of overweight or obese patients.

REFERENCES

1. Aren J, Tsang-Quinn J, Levine C, et al. The Patient Centered Medical Home: components, and review of the evidence. Mt Sinai J Med 2012;79(4):433–50.
2. American Academy of Family Physicians, American Academy of Pediatrics, American College of Physicians, American Osteopathic Association. Joint Principles of the Patient-centered Medical Home. 2007.
3. DeVries A, Li CH, Sridhar G, et al. Impact of medical homes on quality, healthcare utilization, and costs. Am J Manag Care 2012;18(9):534–44.
4. Wexler RK. Patient opinion regarding patient-centered medical home fundamentals. South Med J 2012;105(4):238–41.
5. Lebrun-Harris LA, Shi L, Zhu J, et al. Effects of patient-centered medical home attributes on patients' perceptions of quality in federally supported health centers. Ann Fam Med 2013;11(6):508–16.
6. Nutting PA, Miller WL, Crabtree BF, et al. Initial lessons from the first national demonstration project on practice transformation to a patient-centered medical home. Ann Fam Med 2009;7:254–60.
7. Crabtree BF, Nutting PA, Miller WL, et al. Summary of the national demonstration project and recommendations for the patient-centered medical home. Ann Fam Med 2010;8(Supplement 1):S80–90. S92.
8. Bitton A, Martin C, Landon BE. A nationwide survey of patient-centered medical home demonstration projects. J Gen Intern Med 2010;25(6):584–92.
9. Flegal KM, Carroll MD, Ogden CL, et al. Prevalence and trends in obesity among US adults, 1999-2008. JAMA 2010;303:235–41.
10. Stein CJ, Colditz GA. The epidemic of obesity. J Clin Endocrinol Metab 2004;89: 2522–5.
11. US Preventive Services Task Force. Effectiveness of primary care-relevant treatments for obesity in adults: a systematic evidence review for the US Preventive Services Task Force. Ann Intern Med 2011;155:434–47.
12. US Preventive Services Task Force. Screening for and management of obesity in adults: US Preventive Services Task Force recommendation statement. Ann Intern Med 2012;157(5):373–8.
13. Jensen MD, Ryan DH, Donato KA, et al. Executive summary: guidelines (2013) for the management of overweight and obesity in adults: a report of the American College of Cardiology/American Heart Association Task Force on Practice Guidelines and the Obesity Society published by the Obesity Society and American College of Cardiology/American Heart Association Task Force on Practice Guidelines. Based on a systematic review from the Obesity Expert Panel, 2013. Obesity (Silver Spring) 2014;22(Suppl 2):S5–39.
14. American Academy of Family Physicians. Primary care for the 21st century: ensuring a quality, physician-led team for every patient [Report]. Leawood (KS): American Academy of Family Physicians; 2012. Available at: http://www.aafp.org/dam/AAFP/documents/about_us/initiatives/AAFP-PCMHWhitePaper.pdf.
15. Wadden TA, Volger S, Tsai AG, et al. Review: Managing obesity in primary care practice: an overview with perspective from the POWER-UP study. Int J Obes 2013;37:S3–11.
16. Perri MG, Limacher MC, Durning PE, et al. Extended-care programs for weight management in rural communities: the treatment of obesity in underserved rural settings (TOURS) randomized trial. Arch Intern Med 2008;168(21):2347–54.
17. Harvey-Berino J, West D, Krukowski R, et al. Internet delivered behavioral obesity treatment. Prev Med 2010;51(2):123–8.

18. Bacigalupo R, Cudd P, Littlewood C, et al. Interventions employing mobile technology for overweight and obesity: an early systematic review of randomized controlled trials. Obes Rev 2013;14(4):279–91.

19. Steinberg DM, Tate DF, Bennett GG, et al. The efficacy of a daily self-weighing weight loss intervention using smart scales and e-mail. Obesity (Silver Spring) 2013;21(9):1789–97.

20. Rock CL, Flatt SW, Sherwood NE, et al. Effect of a free prepared meal and incentivized weight loss program on weight loss and weight loss maintenance in obese and overweight women: a randomized controlled trial. JAMA 2010;304(16):1803–10.

21. Donnelly JE, Goetz J, Gibson C, et al. Equivalent weight loss for weight management programs delivered by phone and clinic. Obesity (Silver Spring) 2013;21(10):1951–9.

22. Wadden TA, Butryn ML, Hong PS, et al. Behavioral treatment of obesity in patients encountered in primary care settings: a systematic review. JAMA 2014;312(17):1779–91.

23. Tsai AG, Wadden TA, Rogers MA, et al. A primary care intervention for weight loss: results of a randomized controlled pilot study. Obesity (Silver Spring) 2010;18:1614–8.

24. Wadden TA, Diewald LK, Barg R, et al. A two-year randomized trial of obesity treatment in primary care practice. N Engl J Med 2011;365:1969–79.

25. Wadden TA, Webb VL, Moran CH, et al. Lifestyle modification for obesity: new developments in diet, physical activity, and behavior therapy. Circulation 2012;125:1157–70.

26. Wu WN, Bliss G, Bliss EB, et al. A direct primary care medical home: the Qliance experience. Health Aff 2010;29(5):959–62.

27. Kamerow D. Direct primary care: a new system for general practice. BMJ 2012;345:e4482.

28. Duxbury P. The physician-owned physical therapy department. Orthop Clin North Am 2008;39(1):49–53, vi–vii.

Past, Present, and Future of Pharmacologic Therapy in Obesity

José E. Rodríguez, MD[a],*, Kendall M. Campbell, MD[b]

KEYWORDS

- Obesity • Stimulants • Fat blockers • Antidepressants • Pharmacology treatment

KEY POINTS

- Obesity medications can be classified into 4 categories: fat blockers, antidepressants, stimulants, and diabetes medications.
- Because of cost, most obesity medications are not realistic options for poor and underserved patients.
- Several obesity medications have high abuse potential and should be used with caution.
- None of the current obesity medications are safe for use in pregnant or breast-feeding women.

THE PAST: A BRIEF HISTORY

Medications for obesity treatment have been available for decades. Synthetic thyroid hormone was first used to treat obesity in the 1920s. When used in obese euthyroid patients, patients experience significant side effects associated with hyperthyroidism, such as exophthalmos, hyperthermia, and palpitations.[1] Medications producing rapid fat loss by blocking ATP production in the mitochondria, such as 2 to 4 dinitrophenol (DNP), were used a decade later.[2] Side effects included increased body warmth, sweating, and decreased appetite. More than 100,000 Americans were treated with DNP before it was withdrawn from the market in 1938. Patients who continued to use DNP suffered cataracts and hyperthermia, and premature deaths were reported. DNP is still commercially available and is marketed as a weight loss supplement.[2]

Disclosure Statement: The authors have nothing to disclose.
[a] Department of Family Medicine and Rural Health, The Center for Underrepresented Minorities in Academic Medicine, Florida State University College of Medicine, 1115 West Call Street, #3210 M, Tallahassee, FL 32306, USA; [b] Department of Family Medicine and Rural Health, The Center for Underrepresented Minorities in Academic Medicine, Florida State University College of Medicine, 1115 West Call Street, #3210 N, Tallahassee, FL 32306, USA
* Corresponding author.
E-mail address: Jose.rodriguez@med.fsu.edu

Stimulants, still in use today, appeared on the market in the mid 1930s.[3] Stimulant medications decrease appetite by increasing metabolism, and many forms are still available today. Not all commercially available stimulants have an antiobesity indication. This article reviews only those stimulants currently approved for use in the treatment of obesity.

Simulant use for weight loss has been widespread over the last 6 decades, but not without significant adverse effects. Most notably, the combination of fenfluramine (approved in 1973) and phentermine (approved in 1959) was marketed as Fen-Phen in the 1980s and 1990s. Both medications are stimulant anorectics. Up to 30% of patients who used this medication developed valvular heart disease. Pulmonary hypertension and several deaths were also reported.[4] Fen-Phen was withdrawn from the market in 1997, but phentermine is still commercially available today and is discussed later in this article. Sibutramine, marketed as Meridia or Reductil, is structurally similar to amphetamines and is marketed as an oral anorectic. Sibutramine quickly became popular in the 1990s, but was withdrawn from the US market in 2010, because of an increase in adverse cardiovascular outcomes.[5] Sibutramine subsequently was in some commercially available dietary supplements. Attempts have been made to remove these products from the market.[6]

THE PRESENT: WHAT IS CURRENTLY AVAILABLE

Although the focus of this article is on pharmacologic treatments for obesity, guidelines for non-medication-based interventions exist and are the foundation for treating overweight and obese patients.[7] These guidelines take into account nonpharmacologic approaches to patient care and include surgical options.

Pharmacologic treatment of obesity is indicated for patients with a body mass index (BMI) of 30 or greater, or for patients with a BMI of 27 or greater who have additional comorbidities. The current list of available medications is included in **Table 1**.

Fat Blockers

The pancreatic lipase inhibitor orlistat (Xenical, Alli) is the most well studied of the obesity drugs currently in use.[8] Orlistat was approved in 1999 as a prescription drug. It became available in 2007 as an over-the-counter (OTC) medication. The prescription strength is double the OTC strength. Both formulations are intended to be taken 3 times a day with a fat-containing meal. The generic cost of the OTC preparation averages $59.97 per month. The cost of prescription strength orlistat ranges from $525.33 to $566.00 for a 1-month supply.[9] In one meta-analysis of weight loss drugs

Table 1
Currently available medications for the treatment of obesity

Drug	Availability
Bupropion/Naltrexone (Contrave)	Widely available
Diethylpropion	Schedule IV
Liraglutide	Widely available
Lorcaserin (Belviq)	Schedule IV
Orlistat (Alli, Xenical)	Widely available (OTC)
Phendimetrazine	Schedule III
Phentermine	Schedule IV
Phentermine/Topiramate (Qsymia)	Schedule IV

including 10,631 patients with an average BMI of 36.3 kg/m^2 and average age of 47 years, participants who took orlistat lost 2.9 kg (95% confidence interval [CI] 2.5–3.2) more than those in the placebo arm, a net BMI reduction of 1.1 kg/m^2 (95% CI 1.4–22.3).[10] Three of 4 patients who took orlistat reported gastrointestinal side effects, including fatty/oily stool, increased defecation frequency, liquid stools, fecal urgency, flatulence, flatulence with discharge, or oily evacuation.[11,12] Although readily accessible, orlistat use is not particularly popular among patients because of the side-effect profile.

Antidepressants

The antidepressant combination bupropion/naltrexone (Contrave) is the only antidepressant-containing regimen currently approved for the treatment of obesity. Bupropion increases dopamine activity in the brain, leading to a reduction in appetite and an increase in energy expenditure. Naltrexone blocks opioid receptors, which, when combined with bupropion, is thought to reduce food cravings. Dosing is complicated, involving titration from one daily tablet (90 mg bupropion/8 mg naltrexone) during the first week of treatment to 2 tablets twice daily by the fourth week of treatment. The maintenance dose is typically 360 mg bupropion/32 mg naltrexone daily. Although the individual components of this medication are relatively inexpensive (300 mg bupropion costs $30.07 to $63.25 per month and 50 mg naltrexone costs $37.96 to $102.84 per month), the on-label cost of the combination ranges from $209.60 to $222 per month[9] and is not covered by insurance. Manufacturer's coupons are available to significantly reduce the cost of the first month of treatment. Common side effects of the bupropion/naltrexone combination include nausea (33%), constipation (19%), headache (18%), and vomiting (11%).[12] Contrave is contraindicated in patients with uncontrolled hypertension, an underlying seizure disorder, eating disorders, benzodiazepine or opioid dependence, and in patients who are taking other bupropion-containing products.[11] Four double-blind, placebo-controlled industry-sponsored trials lasting 56 weeks including 4536 patients showed a 5% to 9% weight loss in patients taking bupropion/naltrexone when compared with placebo.[13] Because it is not a controlled substance, and because primary care physicians are familiar with both medications, this medication may increase in popularity. Patients should be informed that this medication can cause a false positive test for amphetamines in urine toxicology screens.

Stimulants

There are currently 4 stimulant medications approved for the treatment of obesity in the United States: diethylpropion, lorcaserin, phendimetrazine, and phentermine. Phentermine is also available in combination with topiramate (Qsymia).

Diethylpropion (tenuate)

Diethylpropion is a central nervous system stimulant similar to bupropion in structure. It is indicated for weight loss and is a schedule IV drug. In a meta-analysis of 13 studies lasting from 6 to 52 weeks, including 80% women who simultaneously received lifestyle treatments, diethylpropion was associated with a 3.0-kg (95% CI 1.6–11.5) weight loss.[14] The most common side effects were constipation, dry mouth, palpitations, headache, insomnia, and elevated blood pressure.[12] Diethylpropion can be taken daily, 1 hour before meals, 25 mg every 8 hours, or as a 75-mg extended release formula. The generic cost ranges from $20.78 to $36.86 per month for thirty 75-mg tablets.[9] Although readily available and relatively inexpensive, it is not a first-line drug for obesity treatment.

Lorcaserin (belviq)

Lorcaserin was approved in 2013 for long-term use in the treatment of obesity. It is a selective 5-hydroxytryptamine receptor 2c agonist and has been listed as a schedule IV drug. It was approved based on 3 premarketing studies, the Behavioral Modification and Lorcaserin for Overweight and Obesity Management (BLOOM), BLOSSOM, and BLOOM DM studies. The BLOOM study followed 3183 obese adults (mean BMI 36.2 kg/m^2) for 2 years.[15] Side effects caused high rates of discontinuation (36%–50%) in this study. Lorcaserin was associated with a dose-dependent weight loss. Patients on placebo lost 0.3 kg, whereas patients on lorcacerin 10 mg once a day lost 1.8 kg. Patients on 15 mg once a day lost 2.6 kg and patients on 10 mg twice a day lost 3.6 kg.[15] This weight loss was statistically significant and dose-related. Lorcacerin is recommended for use in conjunction with lifestyle modification. Potential adverse effects include headache, dizziness, fatigue, nausea, dry mouth, constipation, cough, reduced heart rate, and hyperprolactinemia.[12] Cardiac valvulopathy has been found no more frequently with lorcaserin treatment than with placebo. Lorcaserin should not be used in patients taking selective serotonin reuptake inhibitors (including bupropion), St. John's Wort, or serotonin 5-hydroxytryptamine receptor agonists (sumatriptan, naratriptan, zolmitriptan, rizatriptan, almotriptan, frovatriptan, and elitriptan). Lorcaserin should be used with caution in patients with cognitive impairment, patients with psychiatric disorders, or men with a history of priapism. Lorcacerin is contraindicated for use in pregnant women and nursing mothers.[11]

Most major insurance carriers in the United States do not cover lorcacerin. The cost for typical lorcacerin dosing of 10 mg twice a day ranges from $209 to $221 per month. Manufacturer subsidies are available for eligible patients. A free 15-day medication trial is available from the manufacturer after which patients can receive ongoing assistance with a manufacturer's coupon.[9]

Phendimetrazine (bontril) and phentermine (adipex and suprenza)

Phendimetrazine was first approved for the treatment of obesity in 1959. There are few studies supporting its use. One randomized controlled trial from 1962 included 146 overweight patients, but 36 dropped out. The remaining patients were divided into 4 groups with varying doses of phendimetrazine. The average weight loss for the 4 groups was 3.6 kg. This weight loss is similar to other studies involving phendimetrazine. Patients taking phendimetrazine may experience agitation, changes in libido, blurry vision, dizziness, headache, palpitation, and tachycardia.[12] Phendimetrazine is contraindicated in pregnant and nursing women. Phendimetrazine is available generically in the United States. The monthly cost ranges between $9.35 and $12.68.[9]

Phentermine has been more widely studied than phendimetrazine. A meta-analysis of 9 trials, with an average duration of 24 weeks, showed that participants on phentermine lost more weight compared with those with lifestyle interventions alone (−3.6 kg [95%CI 0.6–6.0]).[14] More than 80% of participants were women, and more than 80% received concurrent lifestyle modification interventions. The meta-analysis indicated that serious adverse events could be as high as 15 per 1000 users. Side effects of phentermine are similar to those of the other stimulants and include tachycardia, increased blood pressure, tremor, dizziness, insomnia, headache, dry mouth, and diarrhea.[11] Phentermine costs range from $12 to $30 per month.

Phentermine/topiramate (qsymia)

The combination of phentermine and topiramate for the treatment of obesity was approved in late 2013. Topiramate has been used as an anticonvulsant and to treat migraine headaches. An incidental finding for patients on topiramate was weight loss. The dosing of phentermine/topiramate also requires titration. Patients generally begin at 3.75 mg/23 mg and increase to 15 mg/92 mg after 6 weeks by doubling the dose bi-weekly. Phentermine/topiramate is a once-daily medication.

The EQUIP study was an early trial of the phentermine/topiramate combination.[16] Patients with an average BMI of 42 were enrolled for 56 weeks. Study participants were randomized into 3 groups: diet and placebo, diet and low-dose phentermine/topiramate (3.75/23 mg), and diet and high-dose phentermine/topiramate (15/92 mg). Dropout rates ranged from 47% in the placebo group to 34% in the high-dose medication group. Participants experienced a dose-related reduction in weight, with 1.6% weight loss in the placebo group, 5.1% in the low-dose group, and 10.9% in the high-dose group.[16]

Side effects are similar to those of phentermine and include paresthesias (20%), dry mouth (19%), constipation (16%), upper respiratory infection (16%), metabolic acidosis (13%), nasopharyngitis (12%), and headache (11%).[12] Some patients also experience the common side effects of topiramate including difficulty concentrating.

Phentermine/topiramate is not covered by most commercial insurance carriers. It is available from $180 to $189 for a 1-month supply of the median dose (7.5 mg/46 mg).[9] Manufacturer's assistance is available to those who qualify.

Diabetes Medications

Liraglutide (victoza , saxenda)

Liraglutide is an injectable, glucagon-like peptide 1 receptor agonist used to treat type 2 diabetes mellitus. It was approved by the US Food and Drug Administration in late 2014 as an obesity treatment. It comes in a multidose, multiple use pen for daily injection. The starting dose is a daily 0.6-mg subcutaneous injection. The dose is increased 0.6 mg every week to a maximum dose of 3 mg daily. Liraglutide can be administered in the abdomen, thigh, or upper arm. The injection site and timing can be changed without significant alterations in pharmacoavailability.

Side effects include nausea (39%), hypoglycemia (23%), diarrhea (21%), constipation (19%), vomiting (16%), and headache (14%). Users also report decreased appetite (10%), dyspepsia (10%), fatigue (8%), dizziness (7%), and abdominal pain (5%). Liraglutide should not be used in patients with a personal or family history of thyroid carcinoma or multiple endocrine neoplasia type 2, because it has been associated with increased risk of medullary thyroid carcinomas.

Liraglutide is covered by many insurance policies for the treatment of type 2 diabetes. Saxenda is considered to be an obesity medication and is, therefore, not usually covered by insurance. The cost of 1 month's treatment ranges from $1087 to $1178.

THE FUTURE

Most current obesity medications are stimulant-based. Newer medications are on the horizon that target different mechanisms of action for the treatment of obesity. Three new medications currently being investigated include beloranib, mirabegron, and gelesis 100.

Beloranib

Beloranib is an injectable medication under investigation for use in the treatment of Prader-Willi syndrome. Beloranib is a methionine aminopeptidase II inhibitor, which reduces hepatic fatty acid production and promotes breakdown of existing fatty acids into glucose. Beloranib is also associated with reduced hunger and food intake. In phase 1b clinical trials, belonarib was associated an average 1 kg per week weight loss in subjects with Prader-Willi syndrome. Associated improvements in cardiovascular risk due to reductions in body fat were also noted.[17] Side-effect and tolerability profiles are pending. Phase 2 clinical trials are underway, and results are expected in 2016.

Mirabegron

Marketed as Myrbetriq as a treatment for overactive bladder, mirabegron was discovered to activate brown fat in rats. When tested in humans, mirabegron was associated with an increase in basal metabolic rate of 40 kcal/d as well as an increase in brown adipose tissue metabolic activity as measured by PET.[18]

Gelesis 100

Gelesis 100 is a proprietary product made from food-grade material that expands in the stomach on consumption; this slows gastric emptying. An industry-sponsored 12-week trial showed that obese subjects who took Gelesis 100 and consumed fewer calories and lost more weight than those on placebo (6.1% on 2.25 g of Gelesis100, 4.5% for 3.75 g of Gelesis 100, and 4.1% on placebo).[19] Another trial showed that obese subjects who took Gelesis 100 consumed less carbohydrates and more protein than those taking placebo ([mean $\pm$ SD] -4.6 ± 9.1 [$P = .003$], -2.9 ± 11.6 [$P = .043$], and 4.7 ± 11.1, with Gelesis 100 2.25 g, Gelesis 100 3.75 g, and placebo, respectively).[20] If approved by the US Food and Drug Administration, Gelesis 100 will be regulated as a medical device.

SUMMARY

Pharmacologic therapy for obesity is one tool in a multifaceted approach to obesity treatment. Over the years, obesity medications have evolved from being mostly stimulant based to newer pharmacologic treatments that work through different mechanisms. Many of these medicines have a variety of indications and are not just used for obesity. In addition to stimulants, current medications block fat uptake or work as antidepressants, and also several are diabetes medications. For maximum benefit, medications need to be part of a comprehensive patient-centered treatment approach to weight loss. Like most therapies, pharmacologic therapies work best when patient adherence is high. Patients who stop taking their antiobesity medications, without proper lifestyle modification, are unlikely to maintain long-term results. Several medications are in the pipeline, further increasing options for patients struggling with the complex problem of obesity.

REFERENCES

1. Halpern B, Halpern A. Why are anti-obesity drugs stigmatized? Expert Opin Drug Saf 2015;14(2):185–9.
2. Grundlingh J, Dargan PI, El-Zanfaly M, et al. 2,4-Dinitrophenol (DNP): a weight loss agent with significant acute toxicity and risk of death. J Med Toxicol 2011; 7(3):205–12.
3. Colman E. Food and Drug Administration's Obesity Drug Guidance Document: a short history. Circulation 2012;125(17):2156–64.
4. Sachdev M, Miller WC, Ryan T, et al. Effect of fenfluramine-derivative diet pills on cardiac valves: a meta-analysis of observational studies. Am Heart J 2002; 144(6):1065–73.

5. Khorassani FE, Misher A, Garris S. Past and present of antiobesity agents: focus on monoamine modulators. Am J Health Syst Pharm 2015;72(9):697–706.

6. Kim JW, Kweon SJ, Park SK, et al. Isolation and identification of a sibutramine analogue adulterated in slimming dietary supplements. Food Addit Contam Part A Chem Anal Control Expo Risk Assess 2013;30(7):1221–9.

7. Jensen MD, Ryan DH, Apovian CM, et al. 2013 AHA/ACC/TOS guideline for the management of overweight and obesity in adults: a report of the American College of Cardiology/American Heart Association Task Force on Practice Guidelines and The Obesity Society. Circulation 2014;129(25 Suppl 2):S102–38.

8. Yanovski SZ, Yanovski JA. Long-term drug treatment for obesity: a systematic and clinical review. JAMA 2014;311(1):74–86.

9. Good Rx. 2015. Available at: http://www.goodrx.com. Accessed May 10, 2015.

10. Padwal R, Li SK, Lau DC. Long-term pharmacotherapy for obesity and overweight. Cochrane Database Syst Rev 2003;(4):CD004094.

11. Seger JC, Horn DB, Westman EC, et al. Obesity Algorithm, presented by the Obesity Medicine Association, 2014-2015. Available at: http://www.obesityalgorithm.org. Accessed May 21, 2015.

12. Medscape Drugs and Diseases. 2015. Available at: http://www.reference.medscape.com. Accessed July 14, 2015.

13. Greig SL, Keating GM. Naltrexone ER/Bupropion ER: a review in obesity management. Drugs 2015;75(11):1269–80.

14. Li Z, Maglione M, Tu W, et al. Meta-analysis: pharmacologic treatment of obesity. Ann Intern Med 2005;142(7):532–46.

15. Smith SR, Weissman NJ, Anderson CM, et al. Multicenter, placebo-controlled trial of lorcaserin for weight management. N Engl J Med 2010;363(3):245–56.

16. Allison DB, Gadde KM, Garvey WT, et al. Controlled-release phentermine/topiramate in severely obese adults: a randomized controlled trial (EQUIP). Obesity (Silver Spring) 2012;20(2):330–42.

17. Zafgen. The Science. 2015. Available at: http://www.zafgen.com/zafgen/our-approach/the-science. Accessed July 14, 2015.

18. Cypess AM, Weiner LS, Roberts-Toler C, et al. Activation of human brown adipose tissue by a β3-adrenergic receptor agonist. Cell Metab 2015;21(1):33–8.

19. 'Smart pill' reduces weight in overweight and obese subjects. ScienceDaily 2014. Available at: http://www.sciencedaily.com/releases/2014/06/140623141859.htm. Accessed July 13, 2015.

20. 22nd European Congress on Obesity (ECO2015), Prague, Czech Republic, May 6-9, 2015: abstracts. Obes Facts 2015;8(Suppl 1):1–272.

Nutritional Therapy

Julie Schwartz, MS, RDN, CSSD, LD

KEYWORDS

- Nutrition therapy • Diet • Fad diets • Healthy eating • Energy deficit
- Macronutrients • Meal replacements • Food

KEY POINTS

- With diligence and attention to dietary detail, significant weight loss and sustainability are possible for many patients.
- The initial goal should be loss of 3% to 5% of body weight over 12 to 16 weeks; a daily caloric deficit of 500 to 750 calories per day is essential to meet this goal.
- In general, most dietary approaches limit added sugars, limit one or more macronutrients (carbohydrates, fat, or protein), eliminate or restrict choices from specific food groups, or replace some meals/snacks with meal replacements for more structured caloric restriction.
- Any dietary changes must take into account individual patient goals, food preferences, resources, and cultural context.
- An interdisciplinary collaboration of nutrition specialists, exercise specialists, and behavioral specialists helps the primary care team meet individual patient's needs.

INTRODUCTION

The prevalence of obesity in the United States has increased alarmingly over the last 30 years.[1] As obesity rates have increased, so has the variety of available treatment options. Some of these treatments are evidence-based and others are more controversial. Easy access to diet and nutrition information has created confusion regarding the best approach to prevention and treatment of obesity. Fortunately, evidence-based guidelines are available for the prevention and treatment of obesity and overweight. This article reviews the following:

- Successful weight loss strategies that improve comorbidity risk factor
- The daily energy deficit needed for recommended rates of weight loss
- The assessment, intervention, and follow-up necessary for weight management and obesity from a nutrition therapy perspective

No conflicts of interest, or funding to disclose.
Department of Defense, MacDill Air Force Base, H: 3613 South Gunlock Avenue, Tampa, FL 33629, USA
E-mail address: jrsagator8@gmail.com

Prim Care Clin Office Pract 43 (2016) 69–81
http://dx.doi.org/10.1016/j.pop.2015.08.012
0095-4543/16/$ – see front matter © 2016 Elsevier Inc. All rights reserved.

- Fad diets and their effectiveness
- The role of food science in treatment and prevention
- The triple threat: fat, sodium, and sugar
- When to use an interdisciplinary team for more comprehensive approaches to weight loss

SUCCESSFUL WEIGHT LOSS

A target weight loss of 3% to 5% of body weight over 12 weeks promotes measurable improvements in metabolic profiles and risk of comorbidities.[2–5] Patients who exhibit this modest amount of weight loss see reduced blood glucose, improved hemoglobin A1c, reduced serum triglycerides, and a lower risk for cardiovascular disease. Weight loss between 5% and 10% of body weight produces additional benefits, including lower blood pressure, an improved lipid profile, and reduced rates of sleep apnea.[2] When patients are successful at losing 3% of total body weight, additional needs can be assessed at follow-up visits. If desired, a new goal of an additional 3% to 5% of body weight loss can be established if needed or desired. The common element of successful weight loss programs centers on an energy deficit of approximately 500 to 750 calories per day. This deficit can be achieved through prescribing a caloric level or restriction of certain types of foods that results in the energy deficit.[2]

Physical activity also creates an energy deficit. The amount of weight lost using physical activity in isolation is more modest. Physical activity does, however, allow additional calories to be consumed while attaining the total deficit needed for weight loss.[2–7] Physical activity is especially helpful for individuals whose caloric needs are low. Nutrition, physical activity, and lifestyle interventions form the bedrock for the prevention and treatment of obesity. Given the diverse expertise required for each of these elements, an interdisciplinary team approach facilitates success for patients interested in significant weight loss.

NUTRITION THERAPY: THE BASICS

A registered dietitian nutritionist (RDN) is uniquely trained and qualified to provide nutrition therapy. RDNs use a stepwise approach to assess individual needs and recommend interventions tailored to each individual patient. Nutrition therapy centers on evidence-based advice to elicit weight loss, improve health indices, and improve overall patient well-being. A comprehensive nutrition assessment can be conducted through consultation with an RDN. By incorporating questions into existing intake or medical history forms, followed by targeted questions during the patient-provider interaction, providers in the primary care setting can address nutrition in a more broad sense, related to weight loss.

As part of your current intake, you may already collect some of the information used to assess nutrition in relation to weight loss. During this first step, pertinent patient history information to obtain includes family and medical history—identifying comorbid conditions, medications, both prescription and OTC (over the counter), height, weight, and waist or abdominal circumference—can be a helpful marker of risk and future success. When working with patients on weight loss, additional information, including weight history to include weight gain and weight loss (include major life events such as graduation, work change, marriage, divorce, moves, and so on), previous diets, or weight loss plans, including medications if applicable, and 24-hour food recall or food frequency. Much of this information can be obtained through incorporating a few additional questions on your intake forms. Metabolic indicators, including lipid profile, serum blood glucose, hemoglobin A1c, vitamin D, and, if otherwise indicated, thyroid markers, are important indicators to assess.

Once you have this information, the second step is assessment of comorbidity risk or diagnosis and body mass index classification (see https://www.nhlbi.nih.gov/health/public/heart/obesity/lose_wt/risk.htm).[6,7] Assessment of meal patterns include frequency of eating out, frequency of convenience food consumption, elimination of food groups, food preferences, use of meal replacements (shakes, bars, frozen or fresh prepared meals), and excessive intake of foods low in nutritional value (sweets, candy, highly processed, or chips), compared with recommendations for healthy eating, such as Dietary Guidelines for Americans. Other indices, including disordered eating patterns and binge eating (regularly consuming unusually large amounts of food and feeling unable to stop or feeling out of control), night eating disorder, and history of disordered eating or eating disorder diagnosis, need to be assessed to ensure that a behavioral health specialist is not integral to your patient's success. Simultaneously, physical activity is incorporated into the assessment: current physical activities, recreational and purposeful exercise, interests and activities enjoyed in the past, and amount of sedentary time daily. Use motivational interviewing, counseling, and coaching skills to assess your patient's knowledge of nutrition and weight loss to include where knowledge was obtained. Ask patient if they want to lose weight and what they would like to learn. Determine motivation to make changes in behavior, not just motivation to lose weight. Use the Transtheoretical Model of Stages of Change (**Fig. 1**).[8] Aid your patient with identifying their motivation to make changes; this can be helpful in identifying the nutrition strategies that will resonate with your patient and may enhance compliance. Ask the importance and confidence of achieving their stated main motivation on a scale of 1 to 10 with 1 being not at all important/confident and 10 being very important/confident. This confidence can help to identify strong motivators for change as well as the challenges that will be present. An RDN would use all of this information to form a nutrition diagnosis, a step unique to the knowledge, skills, and scope of professional practice of the RDN.

The third step is the intervention or recommendations. Begin by taking a nonjudgmental approach with your patient. Guide your patient in healthy eating using many readily available resources, such as MyPlate.gov, the Academy of Nutrition and Dietetics, the American Heart Association (AHA), or the Dietary Approaches to Stop Hypertension (DASH) diet, or refer to the appropriate nutrition plan that will meet their goals, match their food preferences, and meet their time constraints. Recommend 150 to 300 minutes of physical activity per week.[9] If your patient is currently inactive, start slow and encourage the value of 5 to 10 minutes for beginning an exercise

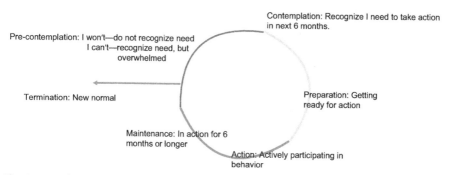

Fig. 1. Transtheoretical model of stages of change.

program. You may want to have a list of local YMCAs (Young Men's Christian Association), certified personal trainers qualified to work with overweight and obese clients, fitness classes, and fitness centers that cater to and have experience working with overweight and obese clients. Technology is constantly evolving, and pedometers, electronic trackers, and other devices can be motivating for many patients.[9] Have the patient set specific goals around 1 to 3 actions, preferably at least one nutrition and one activity goal between visits.

For example, "I will add 2 servings of vegetables to my dinner meal 4 days this week, or I will contact 2 of the resources on your fitness list to learn more about what they offer."

The fourth step is to set up a follow-up session and reassess success based on the goals set at the end of the third step as well as biomarkers. During subsequent appointments, assess percentage of action goals met, weight loss between visits, and total from initial appointment, successes, and the strategies used to reach these successes. Challenges and an action plan to address the challenges when they next arise are part of the process, because challenges and slips will happen with each patient eventually.

Studies indicate the following frequency of visits as most efficacious for weight loss and sustainability[2] of weight loss: initial intervention, weekly for 3 to 6 months; after the initial 3 to 6 months, patient interaction is recommended weekly to bi-weekly for remainder of year. In addition, frequent intervention is recommended at least monthly for up to 2 years.

NUTRITION, DIET FADS, AND TRENDS

Be careful about reading health books. You may die of a misprint.
—*Mark Twain*

Nutrition fads have been around since the 1800s. Many themes have been repeated over the years in these fads (**Fig. 2**). The diet industry generates $60 billion per year. Despite this, since 1996, rates of obesity in the United States have almost doubled. Current data suggest that 36% of US adults (more than 78 million) and 17% (12.5 million) of children (aged 2–19) are obese.

THE QUICK FIX

For many people, fad diets do promote weight loss (**Box 1**). For others, fad diets can jump start the weight loss process, particularly if there is a plan in place to sustain weight loss. For most people, however, any weight lost is quickly regained and often leads to feelings of frustration, failure, or hopelessness.

NUTRITION THERAPY: WHAT DOES THE EVIDENCE SUGGEST?

The evidence suggests that with a daily caloric deficit of 500 to 750 calories multiple approaches work for weight loss.[1] A variety of macronutrient manipulations are efficacious. Some of these are with and some are without formal prescribed energy restrictions. The bottom line with each, however, is a consistent energy deficit. The 2013 American Heart Association/American College of Cardiology/The Obesity Society Guideline for the Management of Overweight and Obesity in Adults[2] provides multiple examples of the types of effective dietary approaches to promote weight loss. One example of weight loss success looked at targeted macronutrient recommendations whereby 15% or 25% of total calories come from protein; 20% or 40% of total calories come from fat, and 35%, 45%, 55%, or 65% of total calories come from carbohydrate, all with a prescribed calorie level creating an energy restriction.

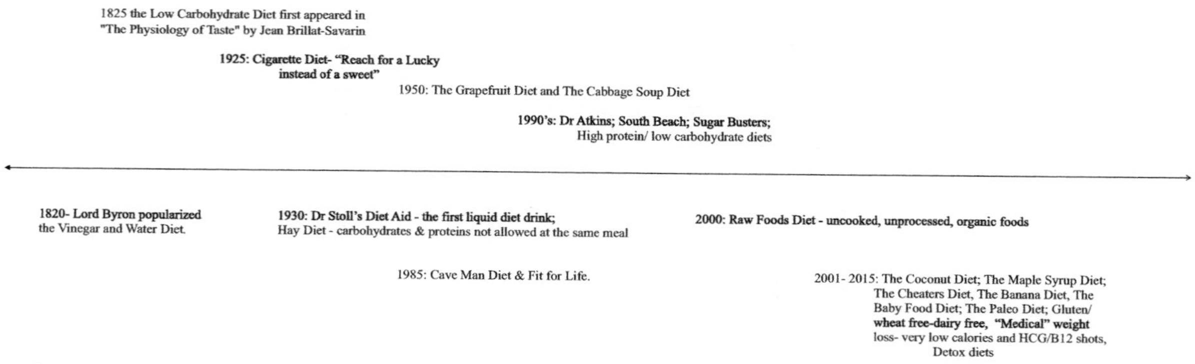

1825 the Low Carbohydrate Diet first appeared in
"The Physiology of Taste" by Jean Brillat-Savarin

1925: Cigarette Diet- "Reach for a Lucky
instead of a sweet"

1950: The Grapefruit Diet and The Cabbage Soup Diet

1990's: Dr Atkins; South Beach; Sugar Busters;
High protein/ low carbohydrate diets

2000: Raw Foods Diet - uncooked, unprocessed, organic foods

2001- 2015: The Coconut Diet; The Maple Syrup Diet;
The Cheaters Diet; The Banana Diet, The
Baby Food Diet; The Paleo Diet; Gluten/
wheat free-dairy free, "Medical" weight
loss- very low calories and HCG/B12 shots,
Detox diets

1820- Lord Byron popularized
the Vinegar and Water Diet.

1930: Dr Stoll's Diet Aid - the first liquid diet drink;
Hay Diet - carbohydrates & proteins not allowed at the same meal

1985: Cave Man Diet & Fit for Life.

Fig. 2. Timeline of Nutrition and Diet Fads. HCG, human chorionic gonadotropin.

Box 1
Diets: Spotting
Consistently promise fast weight loss greater than 2 pounds/week
• Promise little to no effort is needed to lose the weight
• Promise that there is little or no need to exercise
• Eliminate certain food groups
• Require that you purchase pills or supplements that are not US Food and Drug Administration approved to treat obesity
• Tout "superfoods" or specific combinations of foods to boost metabolism
• Rely on personal testimonials instead of scientific evidence

Another example discusses a higher protein option with 25% of total calories coming from protein, 30% of total calories from fat, and 45% of total calories from carbohydrates. Another option promotes 5 meals a day, each with 30% of total calories from protein, 30% of total calories from fat, and 40% of total calories from carbohydrate for realized energy deficit without formal restriction. Patients should focus on targeting food groups instead of formally prescribed restrictions. Patients should lower fat to 30% or less of caloric intake. Foods with a low glycemic load (**Table 1**) have been shown to be effective, however, so have nutrition interventions using a high glycemic load.

Several vegetarian-style diets have been proposed for weight loss. These diets include a lacto-ovo vegetarian diet with a prescribed energy deficit and a low-fat (20% of total calories from fat) vegan diet without formally prescribed energy prescription. Other familiar dietary recommendations include the Mediterranean diet and the AHA Step Diet (**Table 2**).

No one dietary approach is better than another for achieving sustainable weight loss. The best results come from a diet that the patient is able to follow with relative ease and one that fits with their dietary preferences, lifestyle, and cultural context. For example, a patient who is a "carb lover" is going to have difficulty following a pasta-, rice-, or bread-free plan for any length of time. Likewise, a "meat lover" might be challenged to follow a vegetarian diet for any length of time.

Another way to construct an ideal nutritional plan is to tailor dietary recommendations corresponding to the overall health benefits that the patient desires. If, for example, a patient wants to lose weight to improve cardiac health, a diet low in

Table 1	
Low-glycemic-load foods	
Peanuts	Soybeans, cashews
Skim milk	Grapefruit
Orange	Vegetables (carrots, green peas,
Pear, peach	most fresh or canned-in-juice fruits)
Lentils	Legumes—beans (baked, black, kidney)
Whole grain breads—pumpernickel, barley	Couscous
Raisin bran	Yogurt
Oatmeal	Sweet potatoes

Table 2
American Heart Association Step Diet versus new American Heart Association Lifestyle Guidelines versus Mediterranean diet

Step Diet	AHA Lifestyle Guidelines	Mediterranean Diet
<30% calories from fat <1/3 fat calories from saturated fat <300 mg cholesterol/d 6 oz total protein foods/d: emphasis on lean options, such as egg whites, seafood	Know the calorie level appropriate for you to achieve or maintain a healthy weight Limit sodium to 2400 mg/d <30% calories from fat <5–6% total calories Consume fat-free or 1% fat dairy, lean meats, poultry, fish, specifically oily fish containing omega-3 fatty acts (salmon, trout, tuna, herring) twice weekly, nuts, limit red meat Consume fruits, vegetables, whole grains Exercise daily: aim for 30 min of moderate exercise most days of the week Maintain a healthy weight Limit beverages and foods with added sugars Limit alcoholic beverages if you drink	Base every meal on plant-based foods: fruits, vegetables, whole grains, olives and olive oil, beans, nuts, legumes, seeds, herbs, and spices Eat seafood and fish at least twice/wk Consume poultry, eggs, cheese, and yogurt in moderate portions Limit red meat to a few times/mo Enjoy meals with family & friends Be physically active daily

saturated and trans fat will impact cardiovascular health while working toward the weight loss goal if the calorie deficit is also achieved. Currently, most Americans do not consume enough foods that are naturally rich in fiber, such as fruits and vegetables and whole grains. A fiber-rich plan is helpful for treatment of all chronic diseases. Focusing on meal preparation or choosing healthier snack options may be an easier route for some patients.

CREATING A CALORIE DEFICIT

There are a variety of ways to calculate the 500- to 750-calorie deficit depending on patient goals and available resources. A direct measurement of resting metabolic rate (RMR) coupled with calculations of daily energy expenditure is the most accurate. It is also the most labor intensive. Relatively few facilities have the technology to measure RMR. Alternatively, several formulas[3] (**Box 2**) are available to calculate RMR and activity levels. These calculations provide an excellent starting point. Calories can be adjusted depending on the trajectory of weight loss. Many practitioners use a standard daily caloric requirement of 1200 to 1500 calories for women and 1500 to 1800 calories for men. This amount is a reasonable starting point, but often requires significant trial and error that may create frustration for some patients. As patients attempt to lose weight, many will not be exercising at a level of intensity high enough to build muscle mass. Furthermore, it is challenging for the average person's body to be both catabolic and anabolic simultaneously. Therefore, weight gains need to be addressed.

Most evidence indicates that a diet incorporating 25% to 35% calories from fat, higher levels of fiber, with adequate protein and carbohydrates to meet a patients

---

Box 2
Calculating resting metabolic rate or basal metabolic rate

Mifflin-St Jeor

Men: 10 × weight (kg) + 6.25 × height (cm) − 5 × age (y) + 5

Women: 10 × weight (kg) + 6.25 × height (cm) − 5 × age (y) − 161

Multiply by 1.2 to 1.9 for activity.

Institute of Medicine

Men: Basal metabolic rate (BMR; kcal/d) = 293 − (3.8 × age) + (456.4 × height) + (10.12 × weight)

Women: BMR (kcal/d) = 247 − (2.67 × age) + (401.5 × height) + (8.6 × weight)

Age is in years; height is in meters, and weight is in kilograms.
Multiply by 1.2 to 1.9 for activity.

---

energy needs, satiety, and health concerns is ideal.[2] The plan should be simple for the patient to follow, provide resources for overcoming barriers, and provide enough flexibility to adapt to various eating environments that patient will encounter when eating outside of the home or traveling. The MyPlate plan and associated resources is one example of an adaptable plan. Using a positive approach focusing on foods to add instead of foods to not eat may help promote patient adherence. The MyPlate visual aid used with a smaller plate (to aid portion control) is sufficient advice for patients to reduce calories and create an adequate energy deficit for weight loss. An 8- to 9-inch plate is an appropriate plate size for patients. An RDN can further tailor the plan to individual patient needs if available.

SUGAR AND FAT: LIMIT SUGAR, TRANS FATS, AND SATURATED FATS

Trends in nutrition historically have followed a cycle. There is often a food or nutrient that is touted as the biggest problem or the best cure. Despite this, no one food or ingredient can be pinpointed as the cause of or cure for excessive weight gain. Excessive consumption of sugar and fat leads to weight gain. Calorie-dense processed and prepackaged foods, desserts, baked goods, and candies take advantage of this and include sugars and fats in robust combination to appeal to consumer taste buds. Sugars and fats are also hidden in cleverly marketed packages that appear to be a healthy alternative. It is important that patients learn to read nutrition labels and be alert for hidden ingredients that can readily sabotage earnest weight loss efforts.

Sugar, in particular, has recently received significant attention. Excess sugar consumption is not healthy and is linked to overweight and obesity because of excess calories. Added sugar is common in processed foods, baked goods, condiments, candies, and sugar-sweetened beverages, all of which lead to consuming additional calories (**Box 3**). Elyse Powell, Royster Fellow at the University of North

---

Box 3
Sugar by any name is sugar

- Granulated sugar
- Brown sugar
- Raw sugar
- High-fructose corn syrup
- Molasses
- Syrup honey
- Raw honey
- Maltose
- Dextrose
- Fructose
- Agave
- Organic sugar
- Any ingredient ending in "-ose"
- Any syrup

Carolina-Chapel Hill, presented her research at Obesity Week 2014, which showed that despite a slight decline in sugar consumption between 2004 (the peak years) and 2010, overall there has been an increase in added sugars consumed by American adults by more than 30% (228 calories per day in 1977 to 300 calories in 2009–2010). During that same time period, calories from added sugars consumed by children increased by approximately 20% (277–329 calories per day).

Some patients may be confused about recommendations regarding fat consumption. Excess calories in the form of fat quickly add up. Helping patients to choose which fats to eat is important. Saturated fat should be limited and trans fats should be avoided. As an alternative, patients should choose lean animal proteins, vegetable proteins, and low-fat dairy products (skim or 1% if possible). Patients should limit added fat (eg, butter) in cooking and at the table. Patients should limit the use of butter, margarine, gravy, mayonnaise, and salad dressings. Healthy fats should be added to the patient's daily nutrition plan and are available through several natural sources, such as vegetable oils (olive, sunflower, canola, corn, and soy), olives, avocados, nuts and seeds, nut butters, and coldwater fish, such as salmon and tuna. Increasing consumption of these foods as fat sources, while keeping calories in check, adds flavors and textures to dishes and may reduce health risks.

TOOLS FOR SUCCESS
Plant-based Food Approach

Registered dietitian nutritionists

RDNs with expertise in weight management often recommend an individualized plan incorporating a whole-food, plant-based approach to choosing foods for meals and snacks, as this is the approach meeting the recommendations for weight management and prevention and treatment of comorbid conditions.[3] Furthermore, this approach can be an inexpensive approach to chronic disease for physicians to incorporate in their practice as well.[10] A plant-based approach emphasizes consumption of whole foods, including vegetables, fruits, legumes, lentils, nuts, and whole grains. Small amounts of animal- or plant-based proteins and fats are included for balance. A thoughtful plant-based diet contains adequate fiber and safely meets daily nutrient requirements for any comorbidity associated with overweight and obesity. Some plant-based diets use a lower carbohydrate approach that minimizes or eliminates some grains and fruits. For interested patients, tailoring a plant-based diet provides a healthy plan that is satiating and nutrient (rather than energy) dense.

Meal Replacements

Evidence from studies including the Diabetes Prevention Study, the Diabetes Prevention Outcomes Studies, and the Look AHEAD trials indicates that meal replacements in the form of balanced ready-to-drink shakes, prepared frozen or fresh meals, and bars are efficient ways to encourage a caloric deficit.[2,3] A variety of meal-replacement options are available. These options include replacing one meal or snack a day to replacing all but one meal a day. Cost can be a factor for patients interested in this option.

Journaling

Journaling food intake and activity levels helps many patients adhere to their weight loss efforts. Tracking calorie intake, food consumption patterns, and episodes of mindless eating helps identify sources of hidden caloric intake that disrupt the negative energy balance. Journaling helps clients moderate food choices, creates mindfulness around meals, and can be used to track calories consumed and energy expended or hunger/satiety and mood/emotions related to food choices. A wide variety of applications (apps) and Web sites are available to help journaling activities. Be aware that some patients may prefer old-fashioned pen and paper for more consistent journaling. Sharing this information with the health care team provides additional visibility, allowing for adjustments and guidance for maintaining motivation for patient-centered weight-loss goals. Several apps that have been around for awhile, are consistently accurate, free, or reasonably priced, and are user friendly include Loselt, Livestrong, MyFitnessPal, and Fooducate.

Planning Menus and Graphing Weight

A disciplined approach to meal planning helps patients with food selection by providing a daily, weekly, or monthly template for meals. Predeveloped and personalized plans at specific calorie levels are available from a variety of resources, including National Heart Lung and Blood Institute of the National Institutes of Health, My Menutrition, the Pritikin Longevity Center, MyPlate.gov, the US Department of Health and Human Services DASH menu plans, and dashdietoregon.org. Several of these sites also are a rich source of other handouts to aid your patient's success. An RDN can also help develop individual menu plans. For long-term success, patients need to plan satiating and healthy meals that incorporate their favorite foods and take into account their food preferences and that of their family. Most individuals who are successful initiating and maintaining weight loss plan their meals by creating specific shopping lists to ensure that all meal and snack components are available. Shopping lists also help to curb impulse buying that often accompanies a quick trip to the grocery store. Tracking trends in weight helps some patients visualize progress and sustain weight loss.[3] Trends in your patient's weight are easy to miss if not closely monitored.

ADDITIONAL THERAPIES AND THE INTERDISCIPLINARY TEAM

Whether adjunct therapies such as medications and surgery are used, adjunct lifestyle therapies (including nutrition therapy) are critical to successful weight loss and weight loss sustainability.[6] Inviting health practitioners with expertise in nutrition, physical activity, or behavioral health to partner with your practice provides an interdisciplinary context to support patients engaged in an often complex weight loss journey. Engaging patients in group classes or providing individual consultations benefits all involved.

FOLLOW-UP SESSION TOPICS

The following nutrition topics are helpful to include in follow-up conversations with patients as part of an active weight management program. Meal planning, portion control and appropriate servings sizes, uncovering mindless eating, nutritional information — where to find it and who to trust, label reading, and grocery shopping create the backbone of weight loss nutrition information. Addressing eating out and special occasions is helpful all year because patients will have special occasions at least monthly and this proves challenging for many people, especially in the early weeks of their weight loss journey. Cue recognition and elimination, stress and emotional eating, mindful eating and mindfulness, hunger and satiety, dealing with slips and problem-solving round out topics that help patients navigate their busy lives while implementing the knowledge that they are learning. A list of useful tools, such as apps, Web sites, menus, food labels navigation, and one-page handouts associated with these topics, can be useful for some patients. The Web sites listed provide a variety to choose from. If you do not have an interdisciplinary team onsite, a list of practitioners that provide additional expertise is useful.

NUTRITION MANAGEMENT FOLLOWING BARIATRIC SURGERY

During the first 6 to 12 months after bariatric surgery, patients are placed on a dietary protocol to build tolerance to foods, slowly stretch the pouch size, and learn new strategies to eat, which accomplishes these goals and also underlying behaviors that increase food tolerance and weight loss maintenance. Similar to any patient undergoing gastrointestinal surgery, the bariatric patient will begin with a liquid diet and advance as tolerated within a few days to a soft diet. The soft diet is limited in fibrous foods, beef, and raw vegetables, making digestion easier and enhancing food tolerance. The length of time following this phase varies greatly between surgery centers; however, typically it begins within 3 days after surgery, as tolerated. Patients are encouraged to take small bites and chew food well, also to aid digestion and food tolerance,[11] but with the added behavior that will prove beneficial long term. Unique to the bariatric surgery patient during this phase, the patient's stomach pouch is very small; therefore, food quantity is severely limited. This limited food quantity results in a very low-calorie diet and the need for minimal protein requirements of 60 g daily. As volume increases during the first 6 to 12 months, protein needs are recalculated to individual patient needs. Balanced meals are encouraged; however, protein is very satiating, and many patients struggle with this recommendation and minimal protein intake in the early days. Patients are encouraged to meet fluid needs between meals. As tolerance increases, additional foods are added. Many surgery centers also have a stepwise approach to slowly increase the volume of food at each meal/snack to appropriately stretch their patient's stomach pouch.

Six to 12 months after the procedure, the nutrition recommendations after bariatric surgery are similar to weight management advice for any other patient. The only exception involves vitamin and mineral supplementation based on laboratory assessment, food tolerance, and surgery performed.[11]

SUCCESSFUL WEIGHT LOSS: LESSONS LEARNED

The National Weight Control Registry[12] tracks people who have lost significant weight, 30 to 300 pounds, and kept it off for several years. The following are characteristic behaviors exhibited by registry participants. Registry participants lost weight through a wide variety of methods and have all maintained weight loss using a combination of the following strategies:

- Follow a low-calorie, low-fat diet
- Eat breakfast daily—typically a fiber-rich cereal, fruit, and low-fat milk
- Track daily or weekly weight trends
- Limit screen time to less than 10 hours per week
- Engage in physical activity for at least 1 hour every day.

SUMMARY

With diligence and attention to dietary detail, significant weight loss and sustainability are possible for many patients. The initial goal should be loss of 3% to 5% of body weight over 12 to 16 weeks. A daily caloric deficit of 500 to 750 calories per day is essential to meet this goal. Several dietary approaches are effective. In general, most limit added sugars, limit one or more macronutrients (carbohydrates, fat, or protein), eliminate or restrict choices from specific food groups, or replace some meals/snacks with meal replacements for more structured caloric restriction. Any dietary changes must take into account individual patient goals, food preferences, resources, and cultural context. An interdisciplinary collaboration of nutrition specialists, exercise specialists, and behavioral specialists helps the primary care team meet individual patient's needs.

REFERENCES

1. Flegal KM, Carroll MD, Ogden CL, et al. Prevalence and trends in obesity among US adults, 1999-2000. JAMA 2002;288(14):1723–7.
2. Jensen MD, Ryan DH, Apovian CM, et al. 2013 AHA/ACC/TOS guideline for the management of overweight and obesity in adults: a report of the American College of Cardiology/American Heart Association Task Force on Practice Guidelines and The Obesity Society. Circulation 2014;129:S102–38. Available at: http://circ.ahajournals.org/content/129/25_suppl_2/S102.full.pdf+html. Accessed June 15, 2015.
3. Seagle HM, Strain GW, Makris A, et al. Position of the American Dietetic Association: weight management. J Am Diet Assoc 2009;109(2):330–46.
4. Donnelly JE, Blair SN, Jakicic JM, et al. American College of Sports Medicine (ACSM) Position Stand. Appropriate intervention strategies for physical activity, weight loss and prevention of weight regain for adults. Med Sci Sports Exerc 2009;41:459–71.
5. Managing overweight and obesity in adults systematic evidence review from the obesity expert panel, 2013. Available at: NHLBI.gov. Accessed June 15, 2015.
6. Fujioka K. Management of obesity as a chronic disease: nonpharmacologic, pharmacologic, and surgical options. Obes Res 2002;10:116S–23S.

7. National Heart, Lung, and Blood Institute; Aim for a Healthy Weight. Available at: https://www.nhlbi.nih.gov/health/public/heart/obesity/lose_wt/risk.htm. Accessed June 15, 2015.
8. Transtheortical model of stages of change. Available at: www.prochange.com. Accessed June 15, 2015.
9. 2008 Physical Activity Guidelines for Americans. health.gov; Office of Diesease Prevention and Health Promotion. October, 2008;ODPHP Publication No U0036. Available at: http://health.gov/paguidelines/guidelines/. Accessed June 15, 2015.
10. Tuso PJ, Ismail MH, Ha BP, et al. Nutritional update for physicians: plant-based diets. Perm J 2013;17(2):61–6.
11. Aills L, Blankenship J, Buffington C, et al. ASMBS Allied Health Nutritional guidelines for the surgical weight loss patient. Surg Obes Relat Dis 2008;4:S73–108.
12. National Weight Control Registry. Available at: www.nwcr.ws. Accessed June 15, 2015.

Economic Impact of Obesity

Elena A. Spieker, PhD[a,b,*], Natasha Pyzocha, DO[a]

KEYWORDS

- Obesity • Economic impact • United States • Economic cost • Burden • Cost
- Prevention • Primary care

KEY POINTS

- Medical costs associated with obesity range as high as $209.7 billion and account for more than 20% of all annual health care spending in the United States; estimates of the indirect costs from obesity are as high as $66 billion per year, which yield total (direct and indirect) cost outcomes that may exceed $275 billion annually.
- Much of the direct cost of obesity is attributable to treating high-cost comorbidities such as cardiovascular disease ($193–$315 billion) and type 2 diabetes ($105–$245 billion).
- If costs associated with obesity stayed constant and did not increase from 2010 to 2030, savings in medical spending would total $549.5 billion.
- Economists estimate that effective weight reduction could net cost-savings exceeding $610 billion in 20 years and implementation of food taxes would yield medical savings of more than $17 billion.
- The top 3 cost-saving interventions are environmental (including taxation of unhealthy foods and beverages); reduced advertising of unhealthy foods and beverages—particularly to children; and modifying nutrition labeling to better delineate foods that can be eaten in moderation from foods that can be consumed ad libitum.

In North America, two-thirds of US adults are classified as overweight or obese.[1] Overweight and obese individuals incur comorbidities that account for enormous health care expenditures. Medical costs associated with obesity are estimated to be as high as $209.7 billion.[2,3] This amount accounts for more than 20% of annual

Disclosures: The opinions and assertions expressed herein are those of the authors and are not to be construed as reflecting the views of the Uniformed Services University of the Health Sciences, the Department of Defense, or the US Government. The investigators have adhered to the policies for protection of human subjects as prescribed in 45 CFR 46;
Conflict of Interest: None.
[a] Department of Family Medicine, Madigan Army Medical Center, 9040 Fitzsimmons Avenue, Fort Lewis, WA 98431, USA; [b] Department of Medical and Clinical Psychology, Uniformed Services University of the Health Sciences, 4301 Jones Bridge Road, Bethesda, MD 20814, USA
* Corresponding author. Department of Family Medicine, Madigan Army Medical Center, 9040 Fitzsimmons Avenue, Fort Lewis, WA 98431.
E-mail address: eas2612@gmail.com

health care spending in the United States. In 1998, annual direct obesity-related costs in the United States were estimated at $74 billion, a figure that almost doubled to $147 billion by 2008.[3] It is suggested that the 37% increase in obesity rate (from 18% to 25% of the overall population) was a primary driver of cost increases during this time.[3]

Obesity is on the increase largely because of changing economics of food cost[4] and reduced opportunities for physical activity at work, school, and home.[4–6] The increase in obesity prevalence between 1987 and 2001 accounts for 27% (adjusted for inflation) of the increase in total US per-capita health care spending.[7] In 1987, the spending disparity between obese and healthy-weight individuals was 15%. This figure more than doubled by 2001, far out-pacing increases in overall per capita for the same period.[3]

Without corrective action, the costs associated with obesity are expected to increase[8] in parallel with increases in obesity prevalence.[3] In addition, the prevalence and incidence of chronic diseases are predicted to increase concurrently, further adding to obesity-related costs.[9,10] Reducing costs associated with obesity in North America's food-rich environment centers on effective prevention. Although many solutions have been proposed, an economically successful and sustainable strategy has yet to be used on a large scale.

This article reviews the available research on direct and indirect medical costs and future economic trends associated with obesity and weight-related comorbidities. Cost disparities associated with subsets of the population experiencing higher than average rates of obesity are summarized. The positive impact of even modest weight reduction on the economy and individual health is discussed. Potential high-impact solutions are offered, and future directions proposed.

INDIVIDUAL OBESITY SPENDING

The cost of obesity has been examined on an individual[2,3,7,11–13] and national[2,3,12,14–16] level. Each obese individual creates an estimated excess between $1429[3] and $2741[2] in annual medical costs. Obese individuals incur costs that are 42% higher than healthy-weight peers.[17] It is likely that current costs are higher than recent estimates due to rising rates of obese and morbidly obese persons and an elevated incidence of weight-related diseases. Cost increases in recent years are largely attributed to increases in obesity prevalence[3] rather than an increase in costs of medical care. It is likely that if rates of obesity continue to increase, costs will increase in tandem.

NATIONAL OBESITY SPENDING
Key Points

- The United States leads the world in obesity-related spending.
- Obesity-related medical treatment costs between $147 and $210 billion a year, roughly 10% of all annual medical spending (based on 2006 data).

In the United States, obesity was responsible for almost 10% of all medical spending in 2006 (equivalent to $85.7 billion in 2008 dollars). This amount of medical spending was nearly double the 1998 annual estimate of $42 billion (in 2008 dollars; 6% of total health costs).[3] The United States leads the world in obesity-related spending.[2] In countries with lower obesity rates, the obesity-related costs represent 0.7% to 2.8% of annual health care expenditures.[17]

DIRECT AND INDIRECT COSTS OF OBESITY

The cost of excess weight manifests in a variety of ways: from increased medical expenses that are relatively easy to observe and measure (most notably prescription expenditures and inpatient hospital services) to costs that are much less visible (for example, increases in gasoline and equipment costs secondary to excess weight). The direct costs of obesity are associated with the diagnosis and treatment of obesity and weight-related conditions, relevant health care services, and procedures. Indirect costs relate to morbidity and mortality and reflect events such as lost wages secondary to illness or disability and of a loss of future earnings due to premature death.

DIRECT COSTS OF OBESITY
Key Points

- Direct medical costs are 42% higher among obese adults compared with normal weight individuals.
- Medical spending associated with adult obesity approaches $210 billion a year.

There are multiple health care costs associated with the diagnosis and treatment of obesity. Diagnostic costs include laboratory and radiological tests that may be required to diagnose obesity-related diseases. Treatment costs include outpatient or inpatient health services, therapy (drug or nondrug), or surgeries. Direct costs also include physician reimbursement, ancillary, and home nursing services. Because obesity is associated with increased outpatient visits, inpatient hospital stays, and use of pharmacy and radiology services,[18] medical spending is increased in multiple payment arenas. As a result, direct medical costs are 42% higher in obese patients compared with healthy-weight peers.[3]

The risk of hospitalization is higher among people who are obese.[19] Inpatient hospital services currently consume nearly one-third of US health care spending.[19,20] Obese patients require more outpatient visits, have higher annual provider fees (37%), and have higher expenditures for prescription drugs.[3] Between 1998 and 2006, obesity-related spending for all payers increased substantially for inpatient services (46%), outpatient services (27%), and prescription drugs (80%). The percentage of costs attributable to obesity ranges from nearly 6% for noninpatient and 10% for inpatient care (excluding prescription drugs) to 15% of prescription medication costs.[3]

Cost estimations of large-scale problems such as obesity vary by study, making exact figures difficult to determine. As an example, data from Medical Expenditure Panel Surveys (MEPS) underestimate obesity-related costs because institutionalized patients were not included. The National Health Expenditure Accounts (NHEA) dataset includes institutionalized patients, a population who may be in poorer health than the general population and at increased risk for obesity. As a result, MEPS data attributed $86 billion in costs to obesity (2006) compared with NHEA estimates of $147 billion for the same year.[3]

A more recent study compared MEPS using a statistically more accurate instrumental variable approach. This methodology corrects for reporting error by including a biological child's body mass index (BMI) as a surrogate measure for an individual's self-reported BMI. By grouping the overweight with the obese, costs are likely underestimated because overweight does not incur as many additional medical costs as the obese population does, making the instrumental variable method likely more precise.[2] Using this updated method, the 2006 NHEA estimate of $147 billion spent annually on medical costs for obesity was modified to $209.7 billion.[2]

An examination of 16 US studies that estimated the total cost of obesity using retrospective (database, patient-attributable fraction; PAF) and prospective (modeling) cost estimations of medical expenses linked to obesity[21] showed that cost outcomes greatly vary based on study design and method of analysis. Cost estimations are based on numerous medical expenses and each model can only account for so many variables. PAF studies allow for inferences about particular disease burden, which helps plan interventions, but does not provide a total burden of obesity (as database studies do). Database studies allow for examination of disparities in obesity linked to specific population traits (eg, demographics). Modeling studies provide more flexibility in terms of prospective cost forecasts. Predicted costs are extrapolated from existing figures; thus, each method has inherent limitations.[17,21–23]

INDIRECT COSTS OF OBESITY

In addition to the value of medical costs directly associated with the treatment of obesity and its comorbidities, there are numerous nonmedical costs that affect economic productivity.

Key Points

- Estimates of the indirect costs of obesity are as high as $66 billion per year. Total costs (direct and indirect) may exceed $275 billion annually.
- Aggregate obesity-attributable costs among full-time employees total $73.1 billion per year.
- Employers pay $6.4 billion per year for absenteeism and $30 billion per year because of reduced productivity attributed to obesity.
- Indirect costs related to the "built" environment (changes made to accommodate larger Americans–wider bus/plane seats, and sturdier hospital beds, ambulances, and wheelchairs) have an additional social impact.

Obesity impacts the work environment. Decreased productivity due to absenteeism and presenteeism (reduced productivity while at work), elevated costs paid for disability and insurance claims, reduced quality of life, and lost life years from premature mortality are associated with obesity. These indirect costs are estimated to be as high as $66 billion annually.[24]

LOST PRODUCTIVITY

Aggregate obesity-attributable annual indirect medical costs among full-time employees total $73.1 billion.[25] Obese workers have more short- and long-term absences from work than nonobese employees.[26] Productivity losses caused by obesity-related absenteeism in the United States range from $4.3 to $6.4 billion annually.[3,27] Reduced productivity costs employers an estimated $506 per obese worker annually.[28]

EMPLOYMENT/INSURANCE CLAIMS

Medical claims are higher among obese individuals as well. In addition to work day loss, obesity increases the risk of disability and is associated with higher employer's life insurance premiums and workers' compensation claims.[29,30] Obese workers' compensation claims average $51,091 per 100 full-time employees compared with $7503 among healthy-weight workers.[31]

QUALITY OF LIFE

Obesity adversely impacts quality of life.[30] There is some evidence that obesity is associated with lower per person wage and lower household income.[32] This association may result in a higher probability of bankruptcy.[33] Obese individuals are also subject to social stigma and potential discrimination.[34] The number of productive life years is also reduced due to increased mortality associated with excess weight, and life expectancy decreases with rising BMI.[35]

In addition to costs associated with employment and quality of life, there are unique environmental challenges for emergency responders and health care providers. In order to transport obese patients and properly care for them in a hospital setting, sturdier equipment has been developed or modified from pre-existing structures. Supplemental medical equipment, such as beds, wheelchairs, and bedside commodes, is available to accommodate larger patients. In addition, conventional MRI and computed tomographic scanners may have weight limits or size restrictions that become problematic when delivering patient care. Updating or buying these new devices and equipment can be costly to the medical system.

IS OBESITY MORE EXPENSIVE THAN SMOKING?
Key Points

- Obesity exceeds smoking as the most expensive preventable disease.
- Morbid obesity increases medical costs by 50% annually. This amount is double the increase attributable to smoking (20%).

Obesity is surpassed only by tobacco use as the leading actual cause of death in the United States[36] Although obesity does not contribute to more deaths than smoking, it presents a far greater financial burden, adding more than twice ($2741) the cost of smoking ($1300) per person per year to the health care system.[2,36] Obesity, unlike smoking, does not drastically increase mortality. Although inactivity and obesity are independent risk factors for premature mortality, the overall associated costs for comorbid chronic diseases are higher when taking into consideration longer life spans and increased numbers of individuals with obesity. These increased obesity statistics raise health care costs for everyone; this is analogous to the burden of second-hand smoke. Of 30,529 Mayo Clinic adult employees and retirees, smoking added about 20% ($1274) per year to medical costs[37]; an added cost that was similar to obesity. Morbid obesity (defined as a BMI >40 kg/m^2) increased medical costs by 50% ($5530) per year.[37] With this shift in redefining the most expensive preventable disease in the United States, policymakers and private groups are attempting to find solutions to the obesity cost crisis using lessons learned from second-hand smoking.

COMORBIDITY COSTS
Key Point

- Much of the direct cost of obesity relates to treatment of high-cost comorbidities, such as cardiovascular disease (CVD; including hypertension and coronary heart disease; $193.4 billion) and type 2 diabetes ($105.7–$245 billion).

Obesity increases the risk for multiple diseases.[24] Treatment costs for weight-related diseases have risen significantly.[3] In 2000, total costs associated with obesity-related type 2 diabetes, coronary heart disease, hypertension, gall bladder disease, breast cancer, endometrial cancer, colon cancer, and osteoarthritis were estimated to be almost $117 billion per year.[38] Currently, treatment of obesity-related CVD (hypertension and coronary heart disease; $193.4 billion) and type 2 diabetes ($105.7 billion) exceeds total costs for treatment of obesity-related diseases just 15 years ago.[20]

Cardiovascular Disease

Nearly half of all US adults with CVD are obese.[39] More than 75% of hypertension cases are attributable to obesity. The American Heart Association estimates that direct and indirect costs of CVD (including stroke) total $315.4 billion annually.[40]

Type 2 Diabetes

Twenty years ago, 7.8 million Americans were diagnosed with diabetes. This number increased to approximately 29.1 million Americans in 2012 (many of whom are undiagnosed).[41] More than three-quarters (80%) of people with type 2 diabetes are overweight or obese.[41] Cost estimates from 2007 suggest that treatment costs associated with type 2 diabetes exceed $150 billion annually.[42]

FUTURE TRENDS
Key Points

- Two of 3 American adults are overweight or obese.
- The number of obese and morbidly obese individuals is projected to grow to 42% and 11%, respectively, over the next 15 years.
- Obese and morbidly obese patients have higher costs than overweight patients. The rising prevalence of morbid obesity will add substantial direct ($48–$66 billion) and indirect ($390–$580 billion) annual costs to the US health care system.
- By 2030, lost productivity due to obesity could total $580 billion annually and medical costs to treat preventable obesity-related diseases could increase by $48 to $66 billion per year.

Obesity in the United States has tripled since 1960. Morbid obesity has increased 6-fold, to 6% of the population.[1] If obesity continues to increase at current rates, by 2030, 65 million additional American adults will be obese (raising the obesity rate to 42%). The prevalence of morbid obesity will increase to 11%.[43] Even within the United States military, where service members are penalized for exceeding weight standards, there are excess costs[44] due to high rates of overweight male (54%) and female (34%) and obese (12% overall) service members.[45]

By 2030, lost productivity related to obesity could reach $580 billion annually. Medical costs for treatment of preventable obesity-related diseases could increase by $48 to $66 billion per year.[8] If total health care costs due to obesity in the United States double each decade (as expected), obesity-related cost would reach a staggering $860.7 to $956.9 billion per year.[16] If, however, 2010 obesity rates were to stay constant, savings in terms of cost-avoidance would approach $550 billion by 2030.[43]

SPECIAL POPULATIONS
Key Points

- There are considerable cost disparities between obese men and women.
- Direct medical costs are the primary cost driver for obese men.
- Nonmedical costs, including lost wages and absenteeism, are primary cost drivers among obese women.
- Morbidly obese patients are responsible for the highest cost expenditures.

Disparities by Weight Category and Gender

Overall annual costs are much higher for obese and morbidly obese individuals compared with overweight persons.[11] For men and women, the incremental cost of obesity (men: $2646; women: $4879) are much higher than incremental costs of being overweight (men: $432; women: $524). Among overweight persons of both genders, the primary cost driver is direct medical costs, accounting for 80% and 66% of male and female adult costs annually. The annual costs associated with obesity are much lower for men ($2646) than women ($4879).

A more recent estimate[2] using data from nearly 23,000 patients with average BMI of 27 between the ages of 20 and 64 estimated that extra medical spending due to obesity totals $3613 annually for women and $1152 for men. Although estimates vary between studies, the bottom line is that, among women, costs increase as BMI exceeds 30 in large part due to job-related factors that affect the individual (eg, lower wages) and employers/society (eg, absenteeism), whereas medical spending for men does not significantly increase until BMI exceeds 35.[2]

Costs are increased even more among the severely obese (BMI 35 to <40) and morbidly obese (BMI >40). As BMI exceeds 35 kg/m², incremental costs increase significantly.[43] Direct medical costs are 3.5 times higher for moderately obese individuals.[11] Morbid obesity increases medical costs by up to 50%.[35,37] Morbid obesity is associated with an additional $6000 annual per capita spending.[35]

Older Adults

The prevalence of obesity in older adults is high.[46] About 35% of people 65 years and older were obese in 2007 to 2010.[9] Among adults aged 65 to 74, more than 40% are currently obese.[9] By 2050, the number of persons aged 65 and over in the United States is expected to more than double, rising from 40.2 million to 88.5 million.[47]

Approximately 8.5% of annual Medicare spending is directed toward obesity-related health costs.[3] This cost represents $50 billion of the $585 billion in 2013 Medicare spending.[48] Chronic medical comorbidities are more common among obese Medicare beneficiaries[49] and generate more treatment costs.[42] Some estimates predict substantial Medicare costs ranging from $3.4 to $4.7 billion over 10 years for 4% weight reduction among at-risk 60- to 64-year-old adults[50] to gross savings over 10 years of $7446 to $10,126 per capita with a 10% weight loss.[15] Given that Medicare Part D does not currently cover prescription weight-loss medications, Medicare likely bears a disproportionate burden of obesity and weight-related disease costs in the current market.

Children and Adolescents

Nearly 1 in 5 American children are overweight or obese. The direct costs of childhood obesity total $14.1 billion.[51] Rates of childhood obesity are increasing, and obese children become obese adults.[52,53] Current rates of adolescent obesity are projected to incur $45 billion in obesity-related spending among adults aged 35 to 64 between 2020 and 2050.[54]

ESTIMATED SAVINGS: MEDICAL WEIGHT LOSS
Key Points

- Reducing obesity rates by 1% could save $9.5 billion per year.
- Reducing the average adult BMI by 5% could save $29.8 billion in 5 years, $158 billion in 10 years, and $611.7 billion in 20 years.

Obesity increases the risk for costly chronic diseases that often require life-long treatment. Weight loss is one of the most cost-effective strategies for lowering weight-related health care costs.[20,55] A 5% to 10% weight loss significantly reduces the risk associated with obesity-related chronic diseases. It is estimated that each 1 point increase in BMI increases medical costs and pharmaceutical costs by 4% and 7%, respectively.[8] Reduction of obesity by as little as 1% from 2030 forecasts could result in nearly 3 million fewer obese adults and cost-savings of $9.5 billion per year. Reducing the average adult BMI by 5% could save $29.8 billion in 5 years, $158 billion in 10 years, and $611.7 billion in 20 years.[8] The medical savings from 10% weight reduction among obese adults aged 35 to 64 has the potential for lifetime savings on medical care for 5 common obesity comorbidities of $2200 to $5300 per person (equivalent to $3100–$7400 per person in 2013 dollars).[56,57]

SOLUTIONS: FROM PRACTICE TO POLICY
Key Points

- The best chance of reducing costs associated with obesity is with prevention programs and policy change.
- The top 3 cost-saving interventions are environmental (including tax on unhealthy foods and beverages); reduced advertising of unhealthy foods and beverages to children; and modifying nutrition labeling.
- Successful weight-reduction programs could yield net cost-savings of more than $610 billion in 20 years.
- Implementation of selective food taxes could yield medical savings of more than $17 billion.

Primary disease prevention is historically the most cost-effective means to improve health outcomes.[58] The Australian Assessing Cost-Effectiveness trials in obesity[59] and prevention[60] show several (but not all) primary preventive interventions to be cost-effective in the long term for children and adults. One leading intervention was environmental changes,[61] which included taxation of unhealthy foods and beverages. The other leading interventions included reduced advertising of unhealthy foods and beverages to children and modifying nutrition labeling using a traffic light model to delineate foods that can be eaten in moderation from foods that can be consumed ad libitum.[59,60] The most cost-effective nonsurgical strategies for weight loss in the United States (as of 2014 market prices) are Weight Watchers (compared with Jenny Craig and Vtrim) and Qsymia (compared with Lorcaserin and Orlistat).[62] Despite the evidence for these cost-effective programs, only about 4 cents of every dollar spent on health care in the United States goes toward public health and prevention.[63]

Interventions within individual providers offices range from providing patients written prescriptions that emphasize healthy eating habits, regular physical activity, and adequate sleep, to referring patients to health management programs or community resources, such as local YMCA (Young Men's Christian Association) chapters or nutrition counseling. Broader social and policy-based initiatives focus on making healthy, affordable food accessible in all communities, ensuring healthy food and beverage marketing practices.

Historically, regulatory requirements constrain insurers from paying for programs that are not directly delivered by physicians or other licensed medical providers. Traditional fee-for-service models discourage the use of nonclinical resources, including community health workers and counselors. With recent changes in health care reform, multiple public and private insurers have increased coverage for proven community-based programs[50] to reduce obesity rates. The Affordable Care Act (ACA) has led to a proliferation of community programs and workplace incentives to promote weight loss.

Such community-based strategies can be effective. A recent study showed a return of $5.60 for every $1 invested in proven community-based programs to promote physical activity, improve nutrition, and prevent tobacco use. This program netted annual cost-savings of $16 billion annually within 5 years.[64] The ACA encourages Medicare and Medicaid enrollees to engage in weight management programs with their primary care medical homes, potentially making the provider a powerful purveyor of information on cost-savings for the obese patient. Offering covered preventive medical treatment for obesity could improve health care costs and decrease the risk of chronic diseases associated with obesity. If successful, Medicare savings could exceed $5 billion; Medicaid savings could approach $2 billion, and private payers could save $9 billion.[58]

Policy Limitations

Policy is a faster way to enact changes than grassroots prevention programs. Implementation of such programs entails skills training, service infrastructure, and funding.[5] Program-based interventions may have the benefit of being effective or may just provide the opportunity for education. Policy, once enacted, is often more sustainable and less reliant on ongoing support funding.

The American Medical Association (AMA) officially recognized obesity as a disease in 2013, noting its commitment to reducing "the incidence of cardiovascular disease and type 2 diabetes, which are often linked to obesity."[65] According to the ACA, no plan can discriminate based on a medical condition. Medical coverage for obesity is not available in all states, which may make individuals less likely to seek treatment from a health care professional.[66]

Food Taxes and Subsidies

One policy change that has been proposed is a specific food tax. Economists estimate implementation of food taxes would yield medical savings of more than $17 billion. As an example, sugar-sweetened beverages (eg, soda, sweetened teas, sports drinks) are the largest source of excess calories and added sugar[67–69] and perhaps the single largest environmental driver of obesity.[70,71] Sugar-sweetened beverage consumption (around 45 gallons per person in the United States annually) contributes roughly 70,000 additional empty calories to the typical American diet. One model[72] proposes that a nationwide penny-per-ounce excise tax on sugar-sweetened beverages would reduce consumption of sugar-sweetened beverages by 15% among adults aged 25 to 64.[72] This tax could prevent 2.4 million person-years of diabetes, 95,000 coronary heart events, 8000 strokes, and 26,000 premature deaths over the course of a decade. In addition to $13 billion in tax revenue, there would be an additional $17 billion in medical cost-savings.

In isolation, targeted food taxes and subsidies are not likely to drastically change weight outcomes; however, altering food pricing and tax structures represents one potential approach to modifying the obesogenic food environment in modern America.

SUMMARY

Obesity affects individual patients and society alike. Obesity imposes significant external costs on society through health care expenses. Externalities associated with the current obesity epidemic merit appropriate public interventions and policy change. Addressing the negative health effects of secondhand smoke is a reasonable template of externalities with serious health impact that has been addressed successfully through programs and policy. As the number of obese Americans increases, associated health care expenditures will do the same. To meaningfully address the increase in obesity requires involvement at all levels of the health care system. Individual providers can engage patients to reduce or eliminate intake of sugar-sweetened beverages, reduce screen time, and track food and beverage intake. Community programs, Weight Watchers, and Qysmia are cost-effective nonsurgical weight loss options, and bariatric surgery is a viable option for some obese patients. Employers, communities, and insurers can implement workplace incentives and community-based programs to promote activity and healthy eating. Early intervention is vital because obesity continues to affect growing numbers of American youth. Ultimately, broad policy changes that have long-term cost-savings and combat the negative aspects of the modern obesogenic environment are needed to affect more permanent change.

REFERENCES

1. Ogden C, Carroll M, Kit B, et al. Prevalence of childhood and adult obesity in the United States, 2011–2012. JAMA 2014;311(8):806–14.
2. Cawley J, Meyerhoefer C. The medical care costs of obesity: an instrumental variables approach. J Health Econ 2012;31(1):219–30.
3. Finkelstein EA, Trogdon JG, Cohen JW, et al. Annual medical spending attributable to obesity: payer-and service-specific estimates. Health Aff (Millwood) 2009;28(5):w822–31.
4. Swinburn BA, Sacks G, Hall KD, et al. The global obesity pandemic: shaped by global drivers and local environments. Lancet 2011;378(9793):804–14.
5. Ananthapavan J, Sacks G, Moodie M, et al. Economics of obesity–learning from the past to contribute to a better future. Int J Environ Res Public Health 2014; 11(4):4007–25.
6. Finkelstein EA, Strombotne KL. The economics of obesity. Am J Clin Nutr 2010; 91(5):1520s–4s.
7. Thorpe K, Florence C, Howard D, et al. The impact of obesity on rising medical spending. Health Aff (Millwood) 2004;23(Suppl 2):W4–480, 6.
8. Wang YC, McPherson K, Marsh T, et al. Health and economic burden of the projected obesity trends in the USA and the UK. Lancet 2011;378(9793): 815–25.
9. Fakhouri T, Ogden C, Carroll M, et al. Prevalence of obesity among older adults in the United States, 2007–2010. NCHS Data Brief 2012;(106):1–8.
10. Ogden C, Lamb M, Carroll M, et al. Obesity and socioeconomic status in adults: United States, 2005–2008. NCHS Data Brief 2010;(50):1–8.
11. Dor A, Ferguson C, Langwith C, et al. A heavy burden: the individual costs of being overweight and obese in the United States. 2010. Available at: http://www.stopobesityalliance.org/wp-content/themes/stopobesityalliance/pdfs/Heavy_Burden_Report.pdf. Accessed May 24, 2015.
12. Arterburn D, Maciejewski M, Tsevat J. Impact of morbid obesity on medical expenditures in adults. Int J Obes 2005;29:334–9.
13. Thompson D, Edelsberg J, Colditz G, et al. Lifetime health and economic consequences of obesity. Arch Intern Med 1999;159(18):2177–83.
14. Allison DB, Zannolli R, Narayan KM. The direct health care costs of obesity in the United States. Am J Public Health 1999;89(8):1194–9.
15. Thorpe KE, Yang Z, Long KM, et al. The impact of weight loss among seniors on Medicare spending. Health Econ Rev 2013;3(1):7.
16. Wang Y, Beydoun MA, Liang L, et al. Will all Americans become overweight or obese? Estimating the progression and cost of the US obesity epidemic. Obesity (Silver Spring) 2008;16(10):2323–30.

17. Withrow D, Alter DA. The economic burden of obesity worldwide: a systematic review of the direct costs of obesity. Obes Rev 2011;12:131–41.
18. Quesenberry CP Jr, Caan B, Jacobson A. Obesity, health services use, and health care costs among members of a health maintenance organization. Arch Intern Med 1998;158(5):466–72.
19. Weiss AJ, Barrett ML, Steiner CA. Trends and projections in inpatient hospital costs and utilization, 2003–2013: statistical brief #175. Healthcare cost and utilization project (HCUP) statistical briefs. Rockville (MD): Agency for Health Care Policy and Research (US); 2006.
20. Brill A. Health and Economic Benefits of Weight Loss among Obese U.S. Adults. 2014. Available at: http://static1.1.sqspcdn.com/static/f/460582/25269368/1407334355647/MGA_ObesityCoalition+August+2014_WEB.pdf?token=mWeLGPGZl%2FGz2THwf%2Fq%2F5mtExxs%3D. Accessed June 4, 2015.
21. Bierl M, Marsh T, Webber L, et al. Apples and oranges: a comparison of costing methods for obesity. Obes Rev 2013;14(9):693–706.
22. Levy DT, Mabry PL, Wang YC, et al. Simulation models of obesity: a review of the literature and implications for research and policy. Obes Rev 2011;12(5):378–94.
23. Rowe AK, Powell KE, Flanders WD. Why population attributable fractions can sum to more than one. Am J Prev Med 2004;26(3):243–9.
24. Hammond R, Levine R. The economic impact of obesity in the United States. Diabetes Metab Syndr Obes 2010;3:285–95.
25. Finkelstein EA, DiBonaventura M, Burgess SM, et al. The costs of obesity in the workplace. J Occup Environ Med 2010;52(10):971–6.
26. Colditz GA. Economic costs of obesity. Am J Clin Nutr 1992;55(2 Suppl):503s–7s.
27. Cawley J, Rizzo JA, Haas K. Occupation-specific absenteeism costs associated with obesity and morbid obesity. J Occup Environ Med 2007;49(12):1317–24.
28. Gates DM, Succop P, Brehm BJ, et al. Obesity and presenteeism: the impact of body mass index on workplace productivity. J Occup Environ Med 2008;50(1):39–45.
29. Trogdon JG, Finkelstein EA, Hylands T, et al. Indirect costs of obesity: a review of the current literature. Obes Rev 2008;9(5):489–500.
30. Tucker L, Friedman G. Obesity and absenteeism: an epidemiologic study of 10,825 employed adults. Am J Health Promot 1998;12(3):202–7.
31. Burton WN, Chen CY, Schultz AB, et al. The economic costs associated with body mass index in a workplace. J Occup Environ Med 1998;40(9):786–92.
32. Colditz G, Wang Y. Economic costs of obesity. New York: Oxford University Press, Inc; 2008.
33. Guettabi M, Munasib A. The impact of obesity on consumer bankruptcy. Econ Hum Biol 2015;17:208–24.
34. Carr D, Friedman M. Is obesity stigmatizing? Body weight, perceived discrimination, and psychological well-being in the United States. J Health Soc Behav 2005;46(3):244–59.
35. Finkelstein EA. How big of a problem is obesity? Surg Obes Relat Dis 2014;10(4):569–70.
36. Congressional Budget Office. Raising the excise tax on cigarettes: effects on health and the federal budget. 2012. Available at: http://www.cbo.gov/sites/default/files/cbofiles/attachments/06-13-Smoking_Reduction.pdf. Accessed June 4, 2015.
37. Moriarty JP, Branda ME, Olsen KD, et al. The effects of incremental costs of smoking and obesity on health care costs among adults: a 7-year longitudinal study. J Occup Environ Med 2012;54(3):286–91.

38. Department of Health and Human Services. Prevention makes common "cents". 2003. Available at: http://aspe.hhs.gov/pdf-report/prevention-makes-common-cents. Accessed June 4, 2015.

39. Go AS, Mozaffarian D, Roger VL, et al. Heart disease and stroke statistics–2014 update: a report from the American Heart Association. Circulation 2014;129(3): e28–292.

40. American Heart Association. Heart disease and stroke statistics—2014 update. Circulation 2014;129(3):399–410.

41. Centers for Disease Control and Prevention. National Diabetes Statistics Report: estimates of diabetes and its burden in the United States. 2014. Available at: http://www.cdc.gov/diabetes/pdfs/data/2014-report-estimates-of-diabetes-and-its-burden-in-the-united-states.pdf. Accessed June 4, 2015.

42. Dall TM, Mann SE, Zhang Y, et al. Distinguishing the economic costs associated with type 1 and type 2 diabetes. Popul Health Manag 2009;12(2):103–10.

43. Finkelstein EA, Khavjou OA, Thompson H, et al. Obesity and severe obesity forecasts through 2030. Am J Prev Med 2012;42(6):563–70.

44. Spieker EA, Sbrocco T, Theim KR, et al. Preventing Obesity in the Military Community (POMC): the development of a clinical trials research network. Int J Environ Res Public Health 2015;12(2):1174–95.

45. Barlas FM, Higgins WB, Pflieger JC, et al. 2011 Department of Defense health related behaviors survey of active duty military personnel. Fairfax (VA): ICF International; 2013.

46. Centers for Medicare and Medicaid Services. Chronic Conditions among Medicare Beneficiaries, Chartbook, 2012 Edition. Baltimore (MD); 2012.

47. Vincent G, Velkoff V. The next four decades, the older population in the United States: 2010 to 2050. Washington, DC: US Department of Commerce; 2010.

48. Congressional Budget Office. The budget and economic outlook: 2014 to 2024. 2014. Available at: https://www.cbo.gov/publication/45653. Accessed June 12, 2015.

49. American Hospital Association. Are Medicare patients getting sicker? 2012. Available at: http://www.aha.org/research/reports/tw/12dec-tw-ptacuity.pdf. Accessed June 4, 2015.

50. Thorpe KE, Yang Z. Enrolling people with prediabetes ages 60–64 in a proven weight loss program could save Medicare $7 billion or more. Health Aff (Millwood) 2011;30(9):1673–9.

51. Trasande L, Chatterjee S. The impact of obesity on health service utilization and costs in childhood. Obesity (Silver Spring) 2009;17(9):1749–54.

52. Cawley J. The economics of childhood obesity. Health Aff (Millwood) 2010;29(3): 364–71.

53. Serdula MK, Ivery D, Coates RJ, et al. Do obese children become obese adults? A review of the literature. Prev Med 1993;22(2):167–77.

54. Lightwood J, Bibbins-Domingo K, Coxson P, et al. Forecasting the future economic burden of current adolescent overweight: an estimate of the coronary heart disease policy model. Am J Public Health 2009;99(12):2230–7.

55. Wing RR, Lang W, Wadden TA, et al. Benefits of modest weight loss in improving cardiovascular risk factors in overweight and obese individuals with type 2 diabetes. Diabetes Care 2011;34(7):1481–6.

56. Oster G, Thompson D, Edelsberg J, et al. Lifetime health and economic benefits of weight loss among obese persons. Am J Public Health 1999;89(10): 1536–42.

57. MacLean PS, Wing RR, Davidson T, et al. NIH working group report: innovative research to improve maintenance of weight loss. Obesity (Silver Spring) 2015; 23(1):7–15.

58. Trust for America's Health and Robert Wood Johnson Foundation. F as in fat: how obesity threatens America's future. Washington, DC: Trust for America's Health; 2012.

59. Haby MM, Vos T, Carter R, et al. A new approach to assessing the health benefit from obesity interventions in children and adolescents: the assessing cost-effectiveness in obesity project. Int J Obes (Lond) 2006;30(10):1463–75.

60. Vos T, Carter R, Barendregt JM, et al. Assessing cost-effectiveness in prevention (ACE-Prevention): Final report September 2010. 2010. Available at: http://www.sph.uq.edu.au/docs/BODCE/ACE-P/ACE-Prevention_final_report.pdf. Accessed May 14, 2015.

61. Gortmaker SL, Swinburn BA, Levy D, et al. Changing the future of obesity: science, policy, and action. Lancet 2011;378(9793):838–47.

62. Finkelstein EA, Kruger E. Meta- and cost-effectiveness analysis of commercial weight loss strategies. Obesity (Silver Spring) 2014;22(9):1942–51.

63. Trust for America's health. A healthier America: top priorities for prevention. 2010. Available at: http://healthyamericans.org/assets/files/TFAH%202010Top10Priorities DiseasePrevention.pdf. Accessed June 9, 2015.

64. Robert Wood Johnson Foundation. Return on investments in public health: saving lives and money. 2013. Available at: http://www.rwjf.org/content/dam/farm/reports/issue_briefs/2013/rwjf72446. Accessed June 9, 2015.

65. Press release: AMA adopts new policies on second day of voting at annual meeting (press release). Available at: http://www.ama-assn.org/ama/pub/news/news/2013/2013-06-18-new-ama-policies-annual-meeting.page. Accessed June 3, 2015.

66. Morton J. Affordable Care Act and bariatric surgery. Surg Obes Relat Dis 2014; 10(4):571–2.

67. Andreyeva T, Chaloupka FJ, Brownell KD. Estimating the potential of taxes on sugar-sweetened beverages to reduce consumption and generate revenue. Prev Med 2011;52(6):413–6.

68. Bleich SN, Wang YC, Wang Y, et al. Increasing consumption of sugar-sweetened beverages among US adults: 1988–1994 to 1999–2004. Am J Clin Nutr 2009; 89(1):372–81.

69. Wang YC, Bleich SN, Gortmaker SL. Increasing caloric contribution from sugar-sweetened beverages and 100% fruit juices among US children and adolescents, 1988–2004. Pediatrics 2008;121(6):e1604–14.

70. Brownell KD, Frieden TR. Ounces of prevention—the public policy case for taxes on sugared beverages. N Engl J Med 2009;360(18):1805–8.

71. Institute of Medicine. Local government actions to prevent childhood obesity. Washington, DC: National Academies Press; 2009.

72. Wang YC, Coxson P, Shen YM, et al. A penny-per-ounce tax on sugar-sweetened beverages would cut health and cost burdens of diabetes. Health Aff (Millwood) 2012;31(1):199–207.

Impacts of Physical Activity on the Obese

Meshia Q. Waleh, MD

KEYWORDS

- Obesity • Physical activity • Physician counseling • Pedometers

KEY POINTS

- Fewer than half of US adults engage in the recommended 150 minutes per week of moderate-intensity physical activity.
- Physicians who are regularly physically active themselves are more likely to encourage physical activity for their patients with chronic disease.
- Physical activity reduces the risk for developing obesity, cardiovascular disease, type 2 diabetes mellitus, and some cancers.
- Physical activity, along with dietary modification, is a cornerstone of chronic disease management, in particular for obesity, hypertension, hyperlipidemia, and type 2 diabetes mellitus.
- Electronic applications, pedometers, and school-based programs increase adherence to physical activity recommendations.

Physical activity is defined as any bodily movement produced by skeletal muscles requiring energy expenditure. Physical inactivity has been identified as the fourth leading risk factor for global mortality, causing an estimated 3.2 million deaths globally.[1]

More than one-third of the US population is obese, whereas approximately one-third is overweight. According to the Centers for Disease Control and Prevention (CDC), over the past decade this has been an ongoing trend for the total US population where more of the population is increasingly becoming either overweight or obese. There are gradations of weight: underweight, normal, overweight, obese, morbidly obese, and superobese. Underweight is a body mass index (BMI) less than 19 kg/m². Normal weight is a BMI between 19 kg/m² and 24.9 kg/m². Overweight is defined as a BMI of greater than 24.9 kg/m², whereas obesity is defined as a BMI of greater than 29.9 kg/m². Morbid obesity is further defined as a BMI of greater than 39.9 kg/m². Superobesity is a BMI of greater than 49.9 kg/m². There are

The author has nothing to disclose.
Department of Family and Preventive Medicine, University of South Carolina School of Medicine, 3209 Colonial Drive, Columbia, SC 29203, USA
E-mail address: Meshia.waleh@uscmed.sc.edu

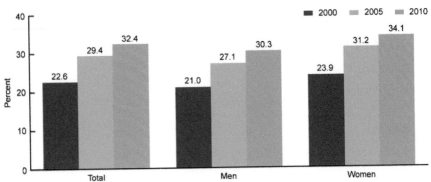

Fig. 1. Percentage of adults aged 18 and over whose physician or other health professional recommended exercise or physical activity, by gender and year: United States—2000, 2005, and 2010. Denominator is adults aged 18 and over who had seen a physician or other health professional in the past 12 months. Age-adjusted to the 2000 US standard population. Access data table for **Fig. 1** at: http://www.cdc.gov/nchs/data/databriefs/db86_tables.pdf#1. (*Courtesy of* Centers for Disease Control and Prevention/National Center for Health Statistics, National Health Interview Survey.)

disproportionately higher rates of obesity in the southern United States and among US minorities (**Figs. 1–6**).

Approximately one-quarter to one-half of physicians recommend weight loss to their patients who are overweight or obese.[2–4] In 2010, approximately one-third (32.4%) of patients reported having been counseled to either increase or begin physical activity by a health professional during the past year.[5]

Less than half of the US population engages in the recommended 150 minutes of weekly moderate-intensity physical activity. Moderate-intensity physical activity is any sustained physical activity that uses 3.5 to 7 calories per minute. Examples of moderate-intensity physical activity include walking at a pace of 3 to 4 miles per

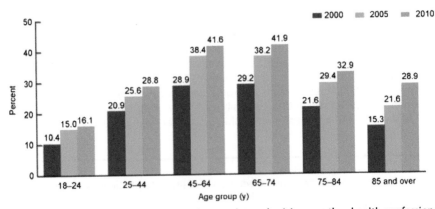

Fig. 2. Percentage of adults aged 18 and over whose physician or other health professional recommended exercise or physical activity, by age group and year: United States—2000, 2005, and 2010. (*Courtesy of* Centers for Disease Control and Prevention/National Center for Health Statistics, National Health Interview Survey.)

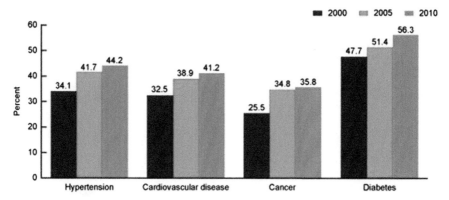

Fig. 3. Percentage of adults aged 18 and over whose physician or other health professional recommended exercise or physical activity, by chronic health condition and year: United States—2000, 2005, and 2010. (*Courtesy of* Centers for Disease Control and Prevention/National Center for Health Statistics, National Health Interview Survey.)

hour, dancing, and gardening. Moderate intensity physical activity expends 3 to 6 metabolic equivalent tasks (METs). METs are a unit of measurement used to quantify intensity of physical activity. METs represent the amount of oxygen that an individual can take in and transport to metabolically active tissues for productive work. They are expressed as a ratio of energy expenditure relative to rest. One MET is equivalent to the amount of energy expended at rest and represents 3.5 mL O_2 per kilogram of body mass per minute.

The 2014 American Time Use Survey showed that only 21% of men and 16% of women were likely to participate in sports, exercise, or recreation on any given day.[6] According to the International Health, Racquet & Sportsclub Association health club industry overview, from 2005 to 2012 the total number of health club members in the United States increased from 41.3 million to 50.2 million. The number of health clubs increased from 26,830 to 30,500 during the same time period.[7] Unfortunately

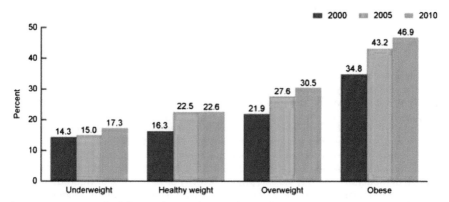

Fig. 4. Percentage of adults aged 18 and over whose physician or other health professional recommended exercise or physical activity, by BMI category and year: United States—2000, 2005, and 2010. (*Courtesy of* Centers for Disease Control and Prevention/National Center for Health Statistics, National Health Interview Survey.)

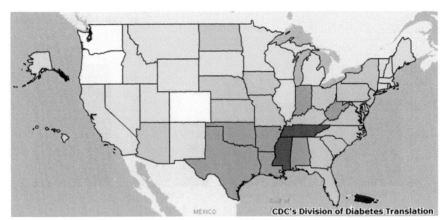

Fig. 5. Age-adjusted leisure-time physical activity percentages. (*Courtesy of* CDC's Division of Diabetes Translation Atlas.)

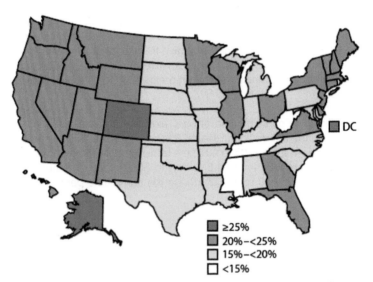

Fig. 6. Proportion of US adults meeting both aerobic and muscle-strengthening physical activity guidelines,* by state—Behavioral Risk Factor Surveillance System, United States, 2011. The figure shows the proportion of US adults meeting both aerobic and muscle-strengthening physical activity guidelines, by state, during 2011. Among the 50 states and the District of Columbia, the prevalence of adults meeting both aerobic and muscle-strengthening guidelines ranged from 12.7% in West Virginia to 27.3% in Colorado.* indicates To meet both the aerobic and muscle-strengthening guidelines from the *2008 Physical Activity Guidelines for Americans*, respondents had to report engaging in at least 150 minutes per week of moderate-intensity aerobic physical activity or 75 minutes of vigorous-intensity aerobic physical activity per week, or an equivalent combination of moderate- and vigorous-intensity aerobic physical activity and participating in muscle-strengthening physical activity at least 2 times per week. (*From* Centers for Disease Control and Prevention. Available at: http://www.cdc.gov/mmwr/preview/mmwrhtml/mm6217a2.htm?s_cid=mm6217a2_e. Accessed June 30, 2015.)

with this growth of health clubs and gym memberships, the number of obese individuals continues to grow in the United States (**Fig. 7**).

REGIONAL VARIATIONS IN OBESITY TRENDS

Discordant regional obesity rates are attributable to, among other factors, a combination of diet, community design, social/cultural norms, and weather. Obesity rates are higher in Southern US states. This is due to a confluence of factors, including employment opportunities, educational opportunities, and access to public trails, regional transportation, food preparation techniques, housing, and health care.[8–11]

The risk of developing obesity depends on multiple factors, including caloric intake and physical activity level. Dietary caloric restriction leads to greater long-term weight loss than exercise. In combination, however, lifestyle modifications, including a controlled, low-calorie diet and increased physical activity, is the most successful intervention for weight loss, weight maintenance, and obesity prevention.[12] All adults should strive for at least 30 minutes of physical activity every day. Smartphone apps and pedometers are available to measure daily steps (the goal is 10,000 steps a day) and provide motivation. Physical activity benefits weight and cardiovascular disease risk. It also has a positive effect on overall health even without a net change in weight.[13] This has been highlighted in individuals with the *FTO* gene variant (conferring a 20%–30% increased obesity risk). In patients with the *FTO* variant, physical activity attenuated obesity by as much as 27%.[14] Overall, moderate-intensity physical activity has a greater effect on reducing cardiovascular mortality than isolated dietary

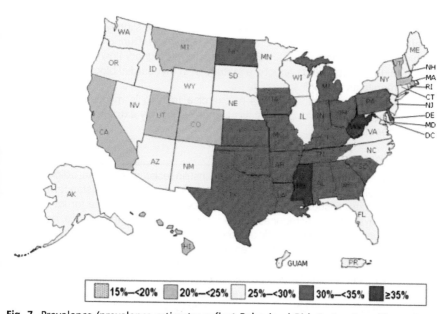

Fig. 7. Prevalence (prevalence estimates reflect Behavioral Risk Factor Surveillance System [BRFSS]) methodological changes started in 2011. These estimates should not be compared with prevalence estimates before 2011 of Self-Reported Obesity among U.S. Adults by State and Territory, BRFSS, 2013. Guam and Puerto Rico were the only US territories with obesity data available on the 2013 BRFSS. (*Courtesy of* Centers for Disease Control and Prevention. Behavioral Risk Factor Surveillance Systems.)

changes, especially for individuals who transition from a sedentary lifestyle to an active lifestyle.

Physical activity should include activities that are enjoyable. Exercising with a partner or a social group also helps incorporate more activity into one's lifestyle.[15] Activity can be done in intervals as short as 10 minutes if target heart rates are achieved. This staggered approach allows for an accumulation of activity throughout the course of a day. An even more simple intervention to reduce obesity risk is to increase the amount of time standing at normally sitting jobs. Research found that those who took advantage of more opportunities to stand at work, take the stairs, and walk to speak with coworkers burned approximately 50 more calories per hour and had a reduction in obesity and type 2 diabetes mellitus rates.[16,17]

EXERCISE PHYSIOLOGY: A BRIEF REVIEW
Cardiovascular Response to Physical Activity

Cardiac output represents the product of stroke volume and heart rate. Heart rate changes in response to sympathetic tone and is the primary component of cardiac output in normal, healthy patients. During exercise, systemic vascular resistance decreases to enhance the delivery of oxygenated blood to exercising muscles. Blood is also shunted away from inactive vascular beds to promote flow to active muscular tissue. During exercise, venous return increases and cardiac contractility goes up in accordance with the Frank-Starling relationship. Increased heart rate and myocardial contractility during exercise combine to increase cardiac output to meet metabolic demands. A normal blood pressure response during exercise is an increase in systolic blood pressure whereas diastolic pressure remains the same or decreases slightly. These proportionate changes in pressure also serve to maximize blood flow to active tissues. During exercise, intrapulmonary pressures increase slightly due to a slight rise in intrathoracic pressure with increased minute ventilation. During exercise, myocardial oxygen demand increases as well. An increase in coronary flow occurs in healthy vasculature. In symptomatic patients, a restriction in myocardial blood flow (coronary ischemia) manifests as angina pectoris.

One of the many beneficial effects of exercise training is myocardial efficiency. When exercised regularly, myocardial tissue more efficiently extracts oxygen for local metabolic needs.

Physical Activity and Glucose Metabolism

Obesity is linked to type 2 diabetes mellitus and insulin resistance. Central adiposity (the deposition of adipose tissue around visceral organs) leads to insulin resistance. In the insulin resistant state, tissues are not able to transport and use glucose for intracellular metabolism. Physical activity reduces insulin resistance, glucose intolerance, postprandial hyperglycemia, and (likely) hepatic gluconeogenesis.[18] Physical activity as an isolated intervention also reduces glycosylated hemoglobin levels by 0.5% to 1%.[18] Physical activity alters the availability of free fatty acids for energy and peripheral fat distribution. Physical activity decreases the amount of abdominal fat in adults regardless of weight loss.[19,20] Numerous adaptive metabolic responses occur with physical training. These adaptations lead to a more efficient oxygen transfer to muscle. Trained muscle is better able use lipid stores as a primary energy source instead of carbohydrates.[21]

Physical Activity and Chronic Disease Reduction

Physical activity reduces cardiovascular risk factors, such as insulin resistance and hypertriglyceridemia. Regular physical activity has also been shown to reduce the incidence of colon cancer and colonic adenomas. Up to at least one-quarter of colon cancer cases could potentially be avoided by lifestyle modifications, including regular physical activity, a healthy diet, and abstaining from tobacco use.[22–24] Physical activity increases cardioprotective high-density lipoprotein levels and reduces circulating triglyceride levels for up to 72 hours postactivity.[18]

INCREASING PHYSICAL ACTIVITY: CAN IT BE DONE?

Physical activity promotes weight maintenance, improves cardiovascular health, and decreases the risk of developing diabetes and cancer. Why then, is it so difficult to motivate many individuals to initiate and sustain programs of regular physical activity? A 2005 Cochrane review evaluated studies examining effective ways to encourage patients to increase the amount of physical activity toward recommended goals. The review analyzed studies that included noninstitutionalized adults aged 16 and older, required a minimum of 6 months of follow-up, used an intention-to-treat analysis, and had no more than 20% loss to follow-up. The review found some interventions either alone or in combination that were moderately successful at increasing the amount of self-reported physical activity and cardiovascular fitness. Those interventions included one-to-one counseling/advice, group counseling/advice, self-directed or prescribed physical activity, supervised or unsupervised physical activity, home-based or facility-based physical activity, ongoing face-to-face support, telephone support, written education/motivational support material, or self-monitoring. Participants still had difficulty achieving recommended daily amounts of physical activity.[25] A more recent 2013 Cochrane Review analyzed 10 studies to assess the effectiveness of face-to-face interventions for increasing physical activity. Inclusion criteria were similar to the 2005 study. Despite study heterogeneity leading to difficulty with broadly generalizing findings, the review found some support for face-to-face interventions as an effective means to increase physical activity for some patients.[26]

Two modalities that may help increase levels of daily physical activity are pedometers and electronic activity monitoring systems. Pedometers are inexpensive and have shown to aid in motivation of daily physical activity. Pedometry has a positive and beneficial influence on quantity of physical activity and helps reduce BMI and blood pressure.[27] Evidence supporting pedometry as a mechanism to increase employee activity is less conclusive.[26] Pedometry can also be useful in helping adults reduce the number of hours seated at their workplace.

Electronic activity monitoring systems are newer wearable technologies that incorporate positive messaging and visual activity aids to promote physical activity goals. Preliminary data indicate that electronic activity monitoring systems help improve physical activity amounts and decrease weight.[28,29] Web-based interfaces and smartphones have also been used to promote activity. A 2013 Cochrane review of 11 moderate and high-quality studies found consistent evidence to support the effectiveness of these newer technology-based interventions. Self-reported physical activity and measured cardiovascular fitness improved at 1 year of follow-up.[29] These results are encouraging because a majority of the US adult population now owns a smartphone. The feasibility and cost-effectiveness across different socioeconomic and ethnic groups remains to be demonstrated. Longer term studies are still needed to determine which modalities, if any, lead to a sustained increase in physical activity levels.

PHYSICAL ACTIVITY—IS IT A ROADBLOCK?

A 2012 survey found that 14% of Americans do not like exercise at all.[15] In the United Kingdom, 6 of 10 individuals would rather die than exercise.[30] The prevalence of automobiles and labor-saving devices discourage physical activity as a routine part of daily life. Lack of physical activity is attributed to more than 5% of disability-adjusted life years. Specifically, inadequate physical activity is most highly linked to diabetes; urogenital, blood, and endocrine disorders; cardiovascular and circulatory diseases; and cancer.[31]

Recently, there has been a suggestion that some cardiac arrhythmias (specifically atrial fibrillation) occur more frequently in elite athletes and those who participate in multiple marathons, ultramarathons, and extreme distance biking races. This suggests that too much physical activity may be harmful. Acknowledging the results of this study, there is little question that the preponderance of evidence supports the beneficial effects of physical activity on cardiovascular health and mortality. When summarizing data for patients who are trying to lose weight, it is likely that elite training does not reduce morbidity and mortality any more than moderate intensity physical activity and in some instances may cause harm.

RESISTANCE TRAINING VERSUS AEROBIC TRAINING

It is well established that resistance training is a central component of any well-rounded activity program. A meta-analysis of 28 studies from 1966 to 1993 revealed that the amount of fat-free mass loss was improved with resistance training compared with weight loss with dietary restriction alone.[29] Weight training helps preserve muscle mass during caloric restriction and weight loss. A systematic review and meta-analysis published in 2015 demonstrated that in individuals who are overfat, resistance training had a positive effect on tumor necrosis factor α, C-reactive protein, leptin, and adiponectin levels. These levels are important markers for cardiovascular disease risk, and a decrease in these levels affords a reduction in negative cardiovascular sequelae.[32,33]

PEDIATRICS

Currently 1 in 6 American children and adolescents is obese. Encouragingly, the rates of obesity in younger Americans seems to have stabilized over the past few years.[34] A 2015 systematic review of 147 articles comprehensively examined the effectiveness of childhood obesity prevention programs. Interventions included school-based programs, school-based programs with a community component, and school-based programs with a home component. Interventions included physical activity alone, diet alone, or a combination of physical activity and diet. Most studies included children between ages 2 and 18 years in developed countries. The results showed high-quality evidence that supports school-based interventions with home involvement that focus on physical activity alone or physical activity with diet if a community aspect is included. Moderate-level evidence supports school-based interventions without a home component that target diet or physical activity alone. Moderate level of evidence also supports interventions that combine physical activity and diet in the school, with community and home components and combined interventions of physical activity and diet in the school or community but without a home component. The evidence highlights the importance of school and community settings in the comprehensive approach to obesity prevention, particularly in children.[35,36]

ADDITIONAL RESOURCES

Additional resources regarding physical activity are listed in **Box 1**.

Box 1
Additional resources

- Fletcher GF, Balady G, Blair SN, et al. Statement on exercise: benefits and recommendations for physical activity programs for all Americans: a statement for health professionals by the committee on exercise and cardiac rehabilitation of the council on clinical cardiology, American Heart Association. Circulation 1996;94:857–62. 8772712.

- Washburn RA, Szabo AN, Lambourne K, et al. Does the method of weight loss effect long-term changes in weight, body composition or chronic disease risk factors in overweight or obese adults? A systematic review. PLoS One 2014;9(10):e109849. Johannsen D, ed. http://dx.doi.org/10.1371/journal.pone.0109849.

- World Health Organization. http://www.who.int/dietphysicalactivity/physical_activity_intensity/en/.

- Funk JL. Disorders of the endocrine pancreas. In: Hammer GD, McPhee SJ, Hammer GD, et al, editors. Pathophysiology of disease: an introduction to clinical medicine. 7th edition. New York: McGraw-Hill; 2013. Available at: http://accessmedicine.mhmedical.com/content.aspx?bookid=961&Sectionid=53555699.

SUMMARY

Prevention of obesity centers on caloric restriction and increased levels physical activity. Weekly physical activity goals should meet or exceed 150 minutes per week of moderate aerobic physical activity. Although many people may not like to exercise, regular physical activity, especially using different modalities and in combination with resistance training, can have an impact on metabolic outcomes, including cardiovascular risk, endocrine diseases, and, importantly, obesity.

REFERENCES

1. Available at: www.who.int/topics/physical_activity/en/. Accessed June 30, 2015.
2. Phelan S, Nallari M, Darroch F, et al. What do physicians recommend to their overweight and obese patients? J Am Board Fam Med 2009;22:115–22.
3. McAlpine DD, Wilson AR. Trends in obesity-related counseling in primary care: 1995–2004. Med Care 2007;45:322–9.
4. Stafford RS, Farhat JH, Misra B, et al. National patterns of physician activities related to obesity management. Arch Fam Med 2000;9:631–8.
5. Barnes PM, Schoenborn CA. Trends in adults receiving a recommendation for exercise or other physical activity from a physician or other health professional. NCHS data brief, no 86. Hyattsville (MD): National Center for Health Statistics; 2012.
6. 2014 American Time Use survey. Available at: http://www.bls.gov/news.release/atus.nr0.htm. Accessed June 30, 2015.
7. Available at: http://www.ihrsa.org/about-the-industry/. Accessed June 30, 2015.
8. Available at: http://content.time.com/time/health/article/0, 8599, 1909406,00.html. Accessed June 30, 2015.
9. Available at: http://livability.com/best-places/top-100-best-places-to-live/2015/ranking-criteria. Accessed June 30, 2015.
10. Available at: Time.com/money/bestplaces. Accessed June 30, 2015.
11. Available at: www.outsideonline.com/1928016/16-best-places-live-us-2014. Accessed June 30, 2015.
12. Available at: http://www.essentialevidenceplus.com.proxy.med.sc.edu/content/eee/154. Accessed June 30, 2015.

13. Shaw KA, Gennat HC, O'Rourke P, et al. Exercise for overweight or obesity. Cochrane Database Syst Rev 2006;(4):CD003817.
14. Kilpeläinen TO, Qi L, Brage S, et al. Physical activity attenuates the influence of FTO Variants on obesity risk: a meta-analysis of 218,166 adults and 19,268 children. PLoS Med 2011;8(11):e1001116.
15. Available at: http://www.heart.org/HEARTORG/GettingHealthy/PhysicalActivity/GettingActive/5-Steps-to-Loving-Exercise-Or-At-Least-Not-Hating-It_UCM_445812_Article.jsp. Accessed June 30, 2015.
16. Available at: http://www.smithsonianmag.com/science-nature/five-health-benefits-standing-desks-180950259/?no-ist. Accessed June 30, 2015.
17. Healy G, Dunstan D, Salmon J, et al. Breaks in sedentary time: beneficial associations with metabolic risk. Diabetes Care 2008;31(4):661–6.
18. Thompson PD, Buchner D, Pina IL, et al. Exercise and physical activity in the prevention and treatment of atherosclerotic cardiovascular disease: a statement from the Council on Clinical Cardiology (Subcommittee on Exercise, Rehabilitation, and Prevention) and the Council on Nutrition, Physical Activity, and Metabolism (Subcommittee on Physical Activity). Circulation 2003;107(24):3109–16.
19. Ross R, Dagnone D, Jones PJH, et al. Reduction in obesity and related comorbid conditions after diet-induced weight loss or exercise -induced weight loss in men: a randomized, controlled trial. Ann Intern Med 2000;133:92–103.
20. Ross R, Janssen I, Dawson J, et al. Exercise-induced reduction in obesity and insulin resistance in women: a randomized controlled trial. Obes Res 2004;12: 789–98.
21. Poirier P, Després JP. Exercise in weight management of obesity. Cardiol Clin 2001;19(3):459–70.
22. Wolin KY, Yan Y, Colditz GA. Physical activity and risk of colon adenoma: a meta-analysis. Br J Cancer 2011;104(5):882–5.
23. Wolin KY, Yan Y, Colditz GA, et al. Physical activity and colon cancer prevention: a meta-analysis. Br J Cancer 2009;100(4):611–6.
24. Erdrich J, Zhang X, Giovannucci E, et al. Proportion of colon cancer attributable to lifestyle in a cohort of US women. Cancer Causes Control 2015;26(9):1271–9.
25. Foster C, Hillsdon M, Thorogood M, et al. Interventions for promoting physical activity. Cochrane Database Syst Rev 2005;(1):CD003180.
26. Richards J, Hillsdon M, Thorogood M, et al. Face-to-face interventions for promoting physical activity. Cochrane Database Syst Rev 2013;9:CD010392.
27. Bravata DM, Smith-Spangler C, Sundaram V, et al. Using pedometers to increase physical activity and improve health: a systematic review. JAMA 2007;298(19): 2296–304.
28. Lewis ZH, Lyons EJ, Jarvis JM, et al. Using an electronic activity monitor system as an intervention modality: a systematic review. BMC Public Health 2015;15:585.
29. Foster C, Richards J, Thorogood M, et al. Remote and web 2.0 interventions for promoting physical activity. Cochrane Database Syst Rev 2013;(9):CD010395.
30. Available at: http://www.theguardian.com/theobserver/2007/sep/23/features.magazine7. Accessed June 30, 2015.
31. Available at: http://www.who.int/healthinfo/global_burden_disease/GlobalHealthRisks_report_full.pdf. Accessed June 30, 2015.
32. Clark JE. Diet, exercise or diet with exercise: comparing the effectiveness of treatment options for weight-loss and changes in fitness for adults (18–65 years old) who are overfat, or obese; systematic review and meta-analysis. J Diabetes Metab Disord 2015;14:31.

33. Garrow JS, Summerbell CD. Meta-analysis: effect of exercise, with or without dieting, on the body composition of overweight subjects. Eur J Clin Nutr 1995; 49(1):1–10.
34. Available at: www.cdc.gov. Accessed June 30, 2015.
35. Wang Y, Cai L, Wu Y, et al. What childhood obesity prevention programmes work? A systematic review and meta-analysis. Obes Rev 2015;16:547–65.
36. Images. National Health Interview Survey, and Behavior Risk Factor Surveillance Systems of the CDC. Available at: www.cdc.gov. Accessed June 30, 2015.

Obesity in Special Populations: Pregnancy

Danielle Symons Downs, PhD

KEYWORDS

• Overweight • Obesity • Pregnancy • Lifestyle modification • Nutrition • Exercise

KEY POINTS

- Perinatal overweight and obesity are associated with multiple maternal and fetal complications, including gestational diabetes, hypertension, macrosomia, and cesarean delivery.
- Maternal obesity and high gestational weight gain are serious public health issues linked to elevated risks for long-term obesity and comorbid diseases in the offspring.
- Preconception assessment and counseling should include a discussion about obesity-related risks and information about proper nutrition, recommended physical activity levels, and perinatal weight management guidance.
- Nutrition and exercise guidance should be offered to all overweight and obese women in the perinatal period.

PERINATAL COMPLICATIONS ASSOCIATED WITH MATERNAL OVERWEIGHT/OBESITY

The average maternal weight at the time of first pregnancy has increased by more than 20% since 1980.[1] Nearly 25% of women presenting for their first prenatal visit now weigh more than 200 pounds and more than 10% of newly expectant mothers exceed 300 pounds.[1] Perinatal overweight and obesity are associated with a number of complications, including gestational diabetes mellitus, hypertensive disorders of pregnancy, cesarean delivery, pulmonary disease, obstructive sleep apnea, and difficulty with anesthesia.[1–3] In addition, overweight and obese women are more likely to exceed recommended perinatal weight gain guidelines (**Table 1** for the Institute of Medicine Guidelines) and keep additional weight on after the delivery.[2] Current data from the Centers for Disease Control and Prevention suggest that excessive weight gain is reported in roughly 59% of overweight women and 56% of obese women,

Support for Dr D.S. Downs for this work has been provided by the National Heart, Lung, and Blood Institute (NHLBI) of the National Institutes of Health through grant SR01HL119245-03.
Exercise Psychology Laboratory, Department of Kinesiology, College of Health and Human Development, Pennsylvania State University, 266 Recreation Building, University Park, PA 16802, USA
E-mail address: dsd11@psu.edu

Table 1 Institute of Medicine recommendations for gestational weight gain	
Weight (BMI [kg/m²])	**Amount of Weight Gain, lbs (kg)**
Underweight (<18.5)	28–40 (13–18)
Normal weight (18.5–24.9)	25–35 (11–16)
Overweight (25.0–29.9)	15–25 (7–11)
Obese[a] (≥30)	11–20 (5–9)

Abbreviation: BMI, body mass index.
[a] Prior guidelines recommended 15 to 25 pounds but this range was dropped to 11 to 20 pounds in 2009.
Data from Institute of Medicine. Weight gain during pregnancy: reexamining the guidelines. In: Rasmussen KM, Yaktine AL, editors. Committee to reexamine IOM pregnancy weight guidelines. Institute of Medicine; National Research Council; 2009. Available at: iom.nationalacademies.org. Accessed November 1, 2015.

and increases the risks for preterm delivery, hypertensive disorders of pregnancy, gestational diabetes, vascular disease, and postpartum weight retention.[3–9]

The rate of overweight and obese women exceeding the gestational weight gain recommendations is predicted to increase in the future owing to the lack of a "gold standard" treatment to prevent high perinatal weight gain. When the 2009 Institute of Medicine report on gestational weight gain[10] was released, there was insufficient evidence to provide weight gain guidelines for women with a body mass index (BMI) of greater than 35 kg/m². Since then, several studies have been published, but the results and recommendations remain equivocal. One large-scale population cohort study[11] suggests that more restrictive weight gain limits in obese women may not harm maternal health or fetal growth. Findings from another study[12] of severely obese pregnant women found the range of gestational weight gain to prevent small- and large-for-gestational-age births may vary by severity of obesity. As a result, the American College of Obstetricians and Gynecologists (ACOG)[13] has stated that an obese woman with an appropriately growing fetus who is gaining less weight than recommended by the guidelines will not experience additional health benefits if she tries to conform with guideline-based weight gain. However, without conclusive evidence from randomized trials, many clinicians are hesitant to recommend that overweight and obese women gain less than the minimum range (ie, 15 pounds for overweight, 11 pounds for obese) recommended by the Institute of Medicine guidelines.[10]

Furthermore, the offspring of overweight and obese women are at increased risk for morbidity and mortality.[10] Multiple fetal complications including premature birth, congenital abnormalities, macrosomia (birth weight of ≥4000 g regardless of gestational age), birth trauma (eg, shoulder dystocia, fracture of clavicle, damage to the brachial plexus) and stillbirth are associated with maternal obesity and excessive gestational weight gain. Women who are obese (BMI >30 kg/m²) are theorized to have elevated circulating levels of insulin (maternal hyperinsulinemia) and a relative state of insulin resistance. According to the "fetal origin of obesity" hypothesis,[14] infants of these obese mothers (or mothers with an excess perinatal weight gain) are exposed to elevated levels of glucose readily crossing the placenta, which leads to a state of fetal hyperinsulinemia and excess fetal growth.[15,16] Maternal obesity more than doubles the risk that a child will become obese by the age of 4 years[17] and this risk is greatest if mothers are obese in the first trimester.[17] Women who are obese at the time of conception are more likely to deliver infants who are not only large-for-gestational age,[18,19] but who also have accelerated weight gain in the first year of life.[20,21] Furthermore, excess maternal weight gain in the first trimester has more influence on infant weight than weight gain in the second and third trimesters.[22]

Evidence also suggests the maternal perinatal metabolic state "programs" metabolism in the fetus. This sets the stage for the trajectory for weight gain during infancy, childhood, and into adulthood. It also predicts risk for obesity, diabetes, and cardiovascular disease[23,24] (**Fig. 1**). Physiologic parameters in the developing embryo and fetus can be "reset" by environmental events (eg, overnutrition, poor glycemic control). These metabolic changes can persist into adulthood to produce a transgenerational nongenetic weight disorder.[24,25]

A child's growth trajectory is governed by control systems based on their genetic constitution and fueled by energy absorbed from the in utero environment.[26] Infants who are born with either a low birth weight (small-for-gestational age) or excess birth weight (large-for-gestational age) are at particular risk for cardiovascular risk and obesity as adults.[27] Excess maternal perinatal weight gain is associated with an large-for-gestational age delivery, regardless of prepregnancy BMI.[28–31] Infants with a birth weight of more than 4000 g have a 2-fold greater risk of adult obesity.[32] On the opposite end of the spectrum are infants who are small-for-gestational age. These infants with a birth weight of less than 2500 g have a 1.9 times greater chance of becoming obese as adults compared with normal birth weight infants. According to the "thrifty genotype" hypothesis, infants exposed to relative malnutrition while in utero are programmed to store nutrients.[20,33] Whether owing to alterations in pancreatic β-cell function or changes in the hypothalamic–pituitary axis,[34] small-for-gestational age infants, when exposed to relative caloric excess outside of the womb, rapidly store calories, gain weight (adiposity rebound),[35] and are at high risk for obesity and cardiovascular disease as adults. When plotted graphically, this represents a U-shaped curve with each end of the curve (small-for-gestational age and large-for-gestational age) being at greater risk for obesity (similar to the phenomenon seen with elderly patients and BMI). Therefore, identifying effective population-level weight management treatment and prevention strategies with capabilities for wide-scale dissemination from conception through adulthood is a critical national priority.

MANAGEMENT OF OBESITY IN PREGNANCY

Managing perinatal overweight and obesity is challenging. Providers must balance the risks of appropriate fetal growth, obstetric complications, and maternal weight gain to

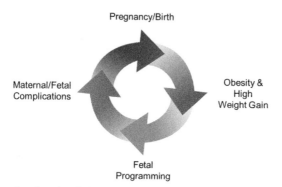

Fig. 1. Intergenerational cycle of obesity.

Table 2
Recommendations for managing obesity in pregnancy

Organization	Recommendations
ACOG[13,36]	• Preconception assessment and counseling are strongly encouraged and should include information on obesity risks and weight loss
	• At initial prenatal visit, record height and weight and calculate BMI (can use online BMI calculator available at www.nilbisupport.com/bmi)
	• Review and discuss gestational weight gain guidelines
	• Discuss appropriate weight gain, diet, and exercise at the initial prenatal visit and periodically throughout pregnancy
	• Nutrition counseling should be offered to all overweight and obese pregnant women and they should be encouraged to follow an exercise program; nutrition and exercise counseling should continue postpartum and before attempting another pregnancy
	• Women who have undergone bariatric surgery should be evaluated for nutritional deficiencies and the need for vitamin supplementation
	• For women who will have a cesarean section who have additional risk factors for thromboembolism, individual risk assessment may require thromboprophylaxis with pneumatic compression devices and unfractionated heparin or LMW heparin
	• Consideration should be given to using a higher dose of preoperative antibiotics for cesarean delivery prophylaxis
	• The use of suture closure of the subcutaneous layer after cesarean delivery in obese patients may lead to a significant reduction in the incidence of postoperative wound disruption
	• Anesthesiology consultation in early pregnancy
	• Individualize care and clinical judgment for the overweight or obese woman who wishes to gain less weight than recommended but has an appropriately growing fetus
	• Consultation with a weight reduction specialist before attempting another pregnancy should be encouraged
IOM[10]	• Organizations should adopt the 2009 weight gain guidelines
	• Health care providers delivering prenatal care should offer them counseling on dietary intake and physical activity that is tailored to their lifestyle circumstances

NHLBI Obesity Education Initiative[37]	• Measure height, weight, and calculate BMI
	• Assess comorbidities
	• Discuss nutrition and physical activity; provide patients with copies of dietary information; encourage goal setting
	• Intervention is based on overall risk assessment
National Institute for Health and Care Excellence[38]	• At first prenatal visit, discuss eating habits and physical activity levels and address any concerns
	• Advise that a healthy diet and physical activity will benefit the woman and her fetus and help her to achieve a healthy weight after birth; advise her to seek information on advice on diet and activity from a reputable source
	• Offer practical and tailored information including how to use increase fruit and vegetable intake
	• Dispel myths about what and how much to eat during pregnancy (eg, no need to "eat for 2" and explain energy needs are only an additional 200 cal/d)
	• Advise that moderate intensity activity will not harm the woman or her fetus and recommend that she achieve 30 min of moderate intensity activity per day
	• Give specific and practical advice about exercising in pregnancy:
	○ Recreational exercise (eg, swimming or brisk walking and strength conditioning) is safe and beneficial
	○ If not a regular exerciser, begin with no more than 15 min of continuous exercise 3 times per week and increase gradually to 30-min sessions; if a regular exerciser before pregnancy, should be able to continue with exercise routine with no adverse effects
	• If women find exercise to be difficult, encourage them to not be sedentary and move more in daily life (eg, take the stairs, reduce sitting for long periods of time)
	• Measure weight and height at first visit and be sensitive to any concerns she may have about her weight; explain importance of actual vs self-reported weight and the need to use this baseline for appropriate weight gain tracking; repeat weighing if clinical management can be influenced or if nutrition is a concern
	• Explain health risks associated with obesity and pregnancy
	• Offer to obese women a referral to a dietician or appropriately trained health professional for assessment and personalized advice on healthy eating and how to be physically active
	• Encourage obese women to lose weight after pregnancy

(continued on next page)

Table 2
(continued)

Organization	Recommendations

Royal Australian and New Zealand College of Obstetricians and Gynecologists[39]	• Identification and management of obesity in the preconceptional period
	  ○ Monitor weight
	  ○ Encourage women to make lifelong and sustainable lifestyle changes
	  ○ Refer to dietician/exercise specialist
	  ○ Meet exercise guidelines
	  ○ Discuss risks of obesity for fertility and pregnancy outcomes, inform women that even modest gain of 1–2 BMI units between pregnancies may increase risks for hypertension, gestational diabetes, and macrosomia
	  ○ If woman has had bariatric surgery, refer to dietician
	  ○ Identification of depressive symptoms
	• Management of obesity in pregnancy
	  ○ Documentation of BMI in pregnancy (women with high BMI should be offered referral to supportive services such as dietician, exercise specialist, etc.)
	  ○ Recommend IOM (2009) guidelines for gestational weight gain and monitor and discuss weight gain consistently throughout pregnancy
	  ○ Recommend to meet exercise guidelines
	  ○ Nutrition supplementation as needed
	  ○ Glucose tolerance testing for gestational diabetes
	  ○ Anesthetic assessment
	  ○ Preeclampsia surveillance
	  ○ Ultrasound assessments of fetal growth
	  ○ Evaluate risk for venous thromboembolism
	  ○ Advise on increased risks of obesity in pregnancy (eg, emergency caesarean section, vaginal delivery [eg, hemorrhage, infant shoulder dystocia])
	• Management of obesity in postpartum
	  ○ Offer support for breastfeeding
	  ○ Offer nutritional and exercise advice following delivery for weight management and weight reduction when applicable

Royal College of Obstetricians and Gynecologists[40]	• All maternity units should have a documented environmental risk assessment regarding availability of resources to care for pregnant women with BMI >30; risk assessment should include: 　o Accessibility including doorway widths and thresholds 　o Availability of properly sized equipment (eg, large blood pressure cuffs, appropriate gown sizes, sit-on weighing scale, large chairs without arms, large wheelchairs, etc) • All health professionals involved in prenatal care should receive education on maternal nutrition and its impact on maternal and fetal health
Society of Obstetricians and Gynecologists of Canada[41]	• Periodic health examinations before pregnancy to offer opportunities to discuss issue of weight loss before conception • Encourage women to enter pregnancy with a BMI <30 and ideally <25 • Counsel women on pregnancy risks associated with obesity and long-term health risks associated with obesity • Obese women should receive counseling about weight gain, nutrition, and food choices • Inform obese women about fetal risks of congenital abnormalities and appropriate screening as applicable • Obstetric care providers should consider BMI for fetal anatomic assessment in second trimester and consider assessment at 20–22 wk for an obese woman • Consultation with anesthesiologist to review options before delivery • Evaluate risk for venous thromboembolism
United State Preventive Services Task Force[42]	• Screen for obesity • Offer referrals to patients with BMI >30 to intensive behavioral interventions

Abbreviations: ACOG, American College of Obstetricians and Gynecologists; BMI, body mass index; IOM, Institute of Medicine; LMW, low molecular weight; NHLBI, National Heart, Lung, and Blood Institute.

optimize fetal outcomes.[13] Because of a deficiency in evidence, there is a lack of standard recommendations for proper management of perinatal obesity. Independent recommendations based on best available evidence from multiple professional organizations are presented in **Table 2**.

The ACOG Committee Opinion on *Challenges for Overweight and Obese Women*[36] highlights multiple factors that can influence women's lifestyles. "Built environmental factors" influencing women's lifestyle in pregnancy are presented in **Box 1**. Other psychological and behavioral factors impacting a woman's likelihood of adhering to recommended lifestyle changes include sociocultural beliefs, levels of motivation and enthusiasm for making and sustaining behavioral changes, behavioral health status (history of anxiety or depression), history of miscarriage or stillbirth, and available support from the patient's social network.[43–45] Another barrier is limited time during routine clinical visits to discuss lifestyle habits and provide adequate counseling about appropriate weight gain, nutrition, and physical activity patterns. Several clinically useful resources for women in the preconceptional, perinatal, and postpartum periods are presented in **Table 3**.

RECOMMENDATIONS

In the absence of widely accepted guidelines for managing overweight and obesity in pregnancy, the following principles apply:

- Measure maternal height and weight at each visit to calculate BMI and track during pregnancy.
- Discuss maternal and fetal health risks associated with excess weight gain and obesity in pregnancy.
- Provide counseling on appropriate weight gain, nutrition, and physical activity.
- Encourage lifestyle and behavioral interventions that are socially and culturally appropriate based on individual patient preference.
- Offer consultation with pain management or anesthesia service for obese women in early pregnancy to have a proactive plan available for labor and delivery.
- Encourage appropriate weight loss before attempting another pregnancy.

The ACOG[36] also recommends that maternity care providers discuss lifestyle modifications with all overweight or obese prenatal patients. Specifically, these conversations at each visit should include discussions about healthy lifestyle behaviors, physical activity, the range of food choices available in local neighborhoods, and safe weight management strategies for pregnancy and the postpartum period.

Box 1
Built environment factors impacting lifestyle

- Access to healthy foods
- Residing in an area with limited grocery stores offering healthy foods at an economical price (also known as a "food desert")
- Easy access to fast food restaurants
- Large portion sizes at restaurants
- Designated areas for safe walking and other physical activities
- Lack of walking paths, trails, or sidewalks
- Lack of access to parks

Table 3
Online resources for managing obesity

Organization	Resource and Website
ACOG	Obesity and pregnancy: www.acog.org/Patients/FAQs/Obesity-and-Pregnancy Weight control: eating right and keeping fit: www.acog.org/Patients/FAQs/Weight-Control-Eating-Right-and-Keeping-Fit Exercise and fitness: www.acog.org/Patients/FAQs/Exercise-and-Fitness
American Obesity Association	Clinical guidelines on the identification, evaluation, and treatment of overweight and obesity in adults: obesity.procon.org/sourcefiles/NIHClinicalGuidelinesObesity.pdf
American Heart Association	Weight management resources: www.heart.org/HEARTORG/GettingHealthy/WeightManagement/Weight-Management_UCM_001081_SubHomePage.jsp
Centers for Disease Control and Prevention	Healthy places and topics: www.cdc.gov/healthyplaces/health_topics.htm Division of Nutrition, Physical Activity, and Obesity resources: www.cdc.gov/nutrition/index.html
NHLBI	NHLBI obesity research: www.nhlbi.nih.gov/research/resources/obesity/ Managing overweight and obesity in adults: www.nhlbi.nih.gov/sites/www.nhlbi.nih.gov/files/obesity-evidence-review.pdf
Shape Up America	Weight, nutrition, and activity resources: shapeup.org/ Pregnancy and weight gain: www.shapeup.org/resources/article_011314.html
USDA Steps to a Healthier You	Choose MyPlate: www.choosemyplate.gov/food-groups/downloads/resource/MyPyramidBrochurebyIFIC.pdf

Abbreviations: ACOG, American College of Obstetricians and Gynecologists; NHLBI, National Heart, Lung, and Blood Institute; USDA, US Department of Agriculture.

Motivational interviewing techniques encourage patients to make a long-term commitment to healthy weight and lifestyle choices. Providers can also sponsor patients for free exercise or wellness programs at local hospitals or health facilities.

SUMMARY

Perinatal overweight and obesity is a major public health and clinical care issue that requires deliberate and immediate attention. Preconception and prenatal assessment and counseling should address the risks associated with obesity, recommendations for weight gain, proper nutrition and dietary intake, and physical activity. Nutrition and exercise guidance should be offered to all perinatal overweight and obese women with an emphasis on effective strategies to overcome barriers. All women should be encouraged to adopt a healthy lifestyle and achieve a healthy weight before becoming pregnant.

REFERENCES

1. Lu GC, Rouse DJ, DuBard M, et al. The effect of the increasing prevalence of maternal obesity on perinatal morbidity. Am J Obstet Gynecol 2001;185(4):845–9.
2. Olson CM, Strawderman MS, Hinton PS, et al. Gestational weight gain and postpartum behaviors associated with weight change from early pregnancy to 1 y postpartum. Int J Obes Relat Metab Disord 2003;27(1):117–27.

3. Flegal K, Carroll M, Kit B, et al. Prevalence of obesity and trends in the distribution of body mass index among US adults, 1999-2010. JAMA 2012;307:491–7.
4. Walker L. Predictors of weight gain at 6 and 18 months after childbirth: a pilot study. J Obstet Gynecol Neonatal Nurs 1996;25:39–48.
5. Gunderson E, Abrams B. Epidemiology of gestational weight gain and body weight changes after pregnancy. Epidemiol Rev 1999;21:261–75.
6. Butte N, Ellis K, Wong W, et al. Composition of gestational weight gain impacts maternal fat retention and infant birth weight. Am J Obstet Gynecol 2003;89:423–32.
7. Ohlin A, Rossner S. Factors related to body weight changes during and after pregnancy: the Stockholm Pregnancy and Weight Development Study. Obes Res 1996;4:271–6.
8. Pirkola J, Pouta A, Bloigu A, et al. Prepregnancy overweight and gestational diabetes as determinants of subsequent diabetes and hypertension after 20-year follow-up. J Clin Endocrinol Metab 2010;95:772–8.
9. Rooney B, Schauberger C. Excess pregnancy weight gain and long-term obesity: one decade later. Obstet Gynecol 2002;100:245–52.
10. Institute of Medicine. Weight gain during pregnancy: reexamining the guidelines: Report brief. In: Rasmussen KM, Yaktine AL, editors. Committee to reexamine IOM pregnancy weight guidelines. Institute of Medicine; National Research Council; 2009. Available at: iom.nationalacademies.org. Accessed November 1, 2015.
11. Beyerlein A, Schiessl B, Lack N, et al. Optimal gestational weight gain ranges for the avoidance of adverse birth weight outcomes: a novel approach. Am J Clin Nutr 2009;90:1552–8.
12. Bodnar L, Siega-Riz A, Simhan H, et al. Severe obesity, gestational weight gain, and adverse birth outcomes. Am J Clin Nutr 2010;91:1642–8.
13. American Congress of Obstetricians and Gynecologists. Obesity in pregnancy. Committee opinion no. 549. Obstet Gynecol 2013;121:213–7.
14. Barker D. Mothers, babies and health in later life. Edinburgh (United Kingdom): Harcourt Brace; 1998.
15. Jolly MC, Sebire NJ, Harris JP, et al. Risk factors for macrosomia and its clinical consequences: a study of 350,311 pregnancies. Eur J Obstet Gynecol Reprod Biol 2003;111(1):9–14.
16. Robinson HE, O'Connell CM, Joseph KS, et al. Maternal outcomes in pregnancies complicated by obesity. Obstet Gynecol 2005;106(6):1357–64.
17. Whitaker RC. Predicting preschooler obesity at birth: the role of maternal obesity in early pregnancy. Pediatrics 2004;114(1):e29–36.
18. May R. Prepregnancy weight, inappropriate gestational weight gain, and smoking: relationships to birth weight. Am J Hum Biol 2007;19(3):305–10.
19. Sebire NJ, Jolly M, Harris JP, et al. Maternal obesity and pregnancy outcome: a study of 287,213 pregnancies in London. Int J Obes Relat Metab Disord 2001; 25(8):1175–82.
20. Baker JL, Michaelsen KF, Rasmussen KM, et al. Maternal prepregnant body mass index, duration of breastfeeding, and timing of complementary food introduction are associated with infant weight gain. Am J Clin Nutr 2004;80(6):1579–88.
21. Li C, Goran MI, Kaur H, et al. Developmental trajectories of overweight during childhood: role of early life factors. Obesity (Silver Spring) 2007;15(3):760–71.
22. Brown JE, Murtaugh MA, Jacobs DR Jr, et al. Variation in newborn size according to pregnancy weight change by trimester. Am J Clin Nutr 2002;76(1):205–9.
23. Heerwagen M, Miller M, Barbour L, et al. Maternal obesity and fetal metabolic programming: a fertile epigenetic soil. Am J Physiol Regul Integr Comp Physiol 2010;299:R711–22.

24. Battsta M, Hivert M, Duval K, et al. Intergenerational cycle of obesity and diabetes: how can we reduce the burdens of these conditions on the health of future generations? Exp Diabetes Res 2011;2011:1–19.
25. Agin D. More than genes: what science can tell us about toxic chemicals, development, and the risk to our children. New York: Oxford University Press; 2010.
26. Tanner J. Growth as a target-seeking function: catch-up and catch-down growth in man. In: Falkner F, Tanner J, editors. Human growth: a comprehensive treatise. 2nd edition. London: Plenum Press; 1986. p. 167–78.
27. McCormick MC. The contribution of low birth weight to infant mortality and childhood morbidity. N Engl J Med 1985;312(2):82–90.
28. Asplund CA, Seehusen DA, Callahan TL, et al. Percentage change in antenatal body mass index as a predictor of neonatal macrosomia. Ann Fam Med 2008; 6(6):550–4.
29. Cogswell ME, Serdula MK, Hungerford DW, et al. Gestational weight gain among average-weight and overweight women–what is excessive? Am J Obstet Gynecol 1995;172(2 Pt 1):705–12.
30. Shapiro C, Sutija VG, Bush J. Effect of maternal weight gain on infant birth weight. J Perinat Med 2000;28(6):428–31.
31. Viswanathan M, Siega-Riz AM, Moos MK, et al. Outcomes of maternal weight gain. Evid Rep Technol Assess (Full Rep) 2008;(168):1–223.
32. Eriksson J, Forsen T, Tuomilehto J, et al. Size at birth, childhood growth and obesity in adult life. Int J Obes Relat Metab Disord 2001;25(5):735–40.
33. Hales CN, Barker DJ. The thrifty phenotype hypothesis. Br Med Bull 2001;60: 5–20.
34. Phillips DI, Barker DJ, Fall CH, et al. Elevated plasma cortisol concentrations: a link between low birth weight and the insulin resistance syndrome? J Clin Endocrinol Metab 1998;83(3):757–60.
35. Rolland-Cachera MF, Deheeger M, Bellisle F, et al. Adiposity rebound in children: a simple indicator for predicting obesity. Am J Clin Nutr 1984;39(1):129–35.
36. American Congress of Obstetricians and Gynecologists. Challenges for overweight and obese women. Committee opinion no. 591. Obstet Gynecol 2014; 123:726–30.
37. US Department of Health and Human Services and National Heart, Lung, and Blood Institute. The practical guide: identification, evaluation, and treatment of overweight and obesity in adults. NIH Publication No. 00–4084. 2000. Available at: www.nhlbi.nih.gov/files/docs/guidelines/prctgd_c.pdf.
38. National Institute for Health and Care Excellence. Weight management before, during, and after pregnancy. NICE public health guidance 27. 2010. Available at: www.nice.org.uk/guidance/ph27. Accessed June 20, 2015.
39. Royal Australian and New Zealand College of Obstetricians and Gynecologists. Management of obesity in pregnancy. College statement C-Obs 49. 2013. Available at: https://www.ranzcog.edu.au/college-statements-guidelines.html. Accessed June 19, 2015.
40. Centre for Maternal and Child Enquiries and Royal College of Obstetricians and Gynaecologists. CMACE/RCOG joint guideline: management of women with obesity in pregnancy. England: CMACE/RCOG; 2010. Available at. www.rcog. org.uk.
41. Davies G, Maxwell C, McLeod L, et al. Obesity in pregnancy. Society of obstetricians and gynaecologists of Canada clinical practice guideline no. 239. Int J Gynaecol Obstet 2010;110(2):167–73.

42. US Preventive Services Task Force. Obesity in adults: screening and management. Available at: www.uspreventiveservicestaskforce.org/Page/Topic/recommendation-summary/obesity-in-adults-screening-and-management. Accessed June 20, 2015.
43. Symons Downs D, Rauff E, Savage J. Falling short of guidelines? Nutrition and weight gain knowledge in pregnancy. J Women's Health Care 2014;3:184–9.
44. Symons Downs D, Devlin C, Rhodes R. The power of believing: salient belief predictors of exercise behavior in normal weight, overweight, and obese pregnant women. J Phys Act Health 2014. http://dx.doi.org/10.1123/jpah.2014-0262. Accessed on June 15, 2015.
45. Symons Downs D, Chasan-Taber L, Evenson K. Obesity and physical activity during pregnancy and postpartum: evidence, guidelines, and recommendations. In: Baptist-Roberts K, Nicholson W, editors. Obesity during pregnancy in clinical practice. New York: Springer; 2014. p. 183–228.

Obesity Statistics

Kristy Breuhl Smith, MD[a],*,
Michael Seth Smith, MD, CAQ-SM, PharmD[b]

KEYWORDS

- Obesity • Obesity epidemic • Epidemiology of obesity • Obesity in adults
- Obesity in children and adolescent

KEY POINTS

- Obesity is a chronic disease that is associated with increased morbidity and mortality, including cancer, cardiovascular disease, disability, diabetes mellitus, hypertension, osteoarthritis, and stroke.
- Obesity occurs because of an energy imbalance between caloric intake and expenditure. The resulting energy excess and associated weight gain are caused by a complex interaction between genetics, environment, economics, and individual behaviors.
- Worldwide, more than 2.1 billion people are overweight or obese. In the United States nearly 35% of adults are classified as obese and one-third of children and adolescents are obese or overweight.
- Overweight and obesity are the fifth leading cause of death in the world, accounting for nearly 3.4 million deaths annually.
- Obesity-related health care costs are difficult to ascertain precisely and vary between countries. In the United States, obesity-related costs of several hundred billion dollars have been reported.

INTRODUCTION

Obesity is a complex, multifactorial disease that is strongly associated with multiple comorbidities.[1–6] These comorbidities include certain types of cancer, cardiovascular disease, disability, diabetes mellitus, gallbladder disease, hypertension, osteoarthritis, sleep apnea, and stroke.[1] Obesity is associated with a high rate of cardiovascular and all-cause mortality.[7] Obesity has been described as a worldwide pandemic.[4] Globally, the prevalence of overweight and obesity increased by 28% in adults and 47% in children between 1980 and 2013.[4] Current estimates suggest that there are nearly 2.1 billion people in the world who are either overweight or obese.[4] In the United

[a] Department of Community Health and Family Medicine, University of Florida, 200 Southwest 62nd Boulevard, Suite D, Gainesville, FL 32607, USA; [b] Department of Orthopedics and Rehabilitation, University of Florida, 3450 Hull Road, Gainesville, FL 32611, USA
* Corresponding author.
E-mail address: kbreuhl@ufl.edu

Prim Care Clin Office Pract 43 (2016) 121–135
http://dx.doi.org/10.1016/j.pop.2015.10.001
0095-4543/16/$ – see front matter Published by Elsevier Inc.

primarycare.theclinics.com

States, data from the National Health and Nutrition Examination Surveys (NHANES) collected between 2011 and 2012 suggest that 35% of adults are obese.[8] Likewise, nearly 17% of American children and adolescents are obese and nearly one-third are either obese or overweight.[8] Obesity is the fifth leading cause of death, estimated to be associated with 3.4 million deaths in 2010.[4] Current trends in obesity seem stable in most developed countries, with the notable exception that the number of individuals classified as morbidly obese continues to increase.[4] The prevalence of obesity in developing countries is increasing toward levels currently seen in the United States.[4] Expenditures of $190 billion per year are associated with the treatment of obesity and obesity-related complications,[9] which represents approximately 21% of total United States health care expenditures.[9] Compared with normal-weight people, obese individuals are responsible for 46% higher inpatient costs, 27% more outpatient visits, and 80% higher spending on prescription medications.[10] Obesity results from an energy imbalance between caloric intake and caloric expenditure. Multiple factors, including genetics, socioeconomic status, environment, and individual decisions, all play a significant role in the pathogenesis of obesity. This article reviews the epidemiology of obesity with an emphasis on disease description, risk factors, prevalence and incidence, and mortalities.

DISEASE DESCRIPTION

To understand obesity, a description of body weight classification for both adults and children is necessary. Body mass index (BMI) is the most widely used standard for classifying somatotype. BMI is obtained by dividing weight in kilograms by height in meters squared. BMI classifications for white, Hispanic, and African American adults have been endorsed by the National Heart, Lung, and Blood Institute, the World Health Organization (WHO), the American Heart Association, American College of Cardiology, and The Obesity Society[2,11,12] (**Table 1**).

- Normal weight: BMI greater than 18 to 24.9 kg/m^2
- Overweight: BMI greater than 25 to 29.9 kg/m^2
- Obesity: BMI greater than 30 kg/m^2
- Obesity class I: BMI of 30 to 34.9 kg/m^2
- Obesity class II: BMI of 35 to 39.9 kg/m^2
- Obesity class III (severe obesity): BMI greater than 40 kg/m^2 (or >35 kg/m^2 in the presence of comorbidities)

This traditional BMI classification underestimates risk in Asian and South Asian people. A separate guideline for this population classifies overweight as a BMI between 23 and 24.9 kg/m^2 and obesity as a BMI of greater than 25 kg/m^2.[13]

Body weight classifications also differ significantly between adults and children because of variations in growth and resultant body surface area. There are also significant differences between boys and girls. The WHO Child Growth Standards are used internationally for children from birth to 5 years old.[1] Updated classifications for children from the age of 5 years old to 19 years old were published in 2007.[1] In the United States, data from the National Center for Health Care Statistics and the Centers for Disease Control and Prevention (CDC) are used to determine age-appropriate weight for children between 2 and 19 years of age (see **Table 1**):

- Normal weight: BMI between the 5th and 85th percentiles for age and sex
- Overweight: BMI between the 85th and 95th percentiles for age and sex
- Obese: BMI greater than 95th percentile for age and sex

Table 1
Common classifications of body weight in adults and children

	Age	Indicator	Normal Weight	Overweight	Obese
Adults	≥20 y	BMI (kg/m²)	18.50–24.99	≥25.00	≥30.00 Class 1: 30.00–34.99 Class 2: 35.00–39.99 Class 3: ≥40.00
Children					
International					
WHO 2006	0–60 mo	BMI Z or WH Z	>–2 to ≤2 SD At risk of overweight: >1 to ≤2 SD	>2 to ≤3 SD	>3 SD
WHO 2007	5–19 y	BMI Z	>–2 to ≤1 SD	>1 to ≤2 SD	>2 SD
IOTF	2–18 y	Growth curve for BMI at age 18	—	BMI = 25	BMI = 30
United States	2–19 y	BMI percentile	≥5th to <85th	≥85th to <95th	≥95th

Abbreviations: IOTF, International Obesity Task Force; SD, standard deviation; WH, weight for height; Z, z score.
Adapted from Hruby A, Hu FB. The epidemiology of obesity: a big picture. Pharmacoeconomics 2015;33(7):674.

- Severe obesity: BMI greater than the 120th percentile or BMI greater than 35 kg/m² (whichever is lower)

For children less than 2 years of age, the CDC recommends using the WHO classifications to determine age-appropriate body weight.[14]

Energy balance, which determines body weight, represents the difference between energy intake and energy expenditure.[15] To maintain a stable body weight, energy intake must equal energy expenditure. Weight gain occurs when energy intake exceeds energy expenditure, resulting in a positive energy balance. Likewise, weight loss occurs when energy expenditure exceeds energy intake. Energy is expended through physical activity and through homeostatic metabolic processes.[15] Although low energy expenditure is one component of excess weight gain, multiple other factors play a significant role. These factors include genetic predisposition, physical inactivity and sedentary behaviors, diet, socioeconomic factors, and other novel risk factors.

RISK FACTORS
Genetics

Obesity occurs when a sustained positive energy balance leads to an increase in body weight. Multiple genetic, social, economic, and personal factors affect this energy balance and the development and maintenance of overweight and obesity. Genetic factors are the only risk factors that are not personally modifiable (**Box 1**).

Family studies including twins and adoptees clearly implicate genetic factors as central to the development of overweight and obesity.[16,17] Studies show a similar risk of obesity in twins raised in separate environments compared with those raised in the same household.[16] Adoptees have been shown to mirror the BMIs of their biological parents rather than their adoptive parents.[16] Although multiple genetic markers have been identified, the 32 most common genetic variants associated with obesity are responsible for less than 1.5% of the overall interindividual variation in BMI.[18]

Box 1
Risk factors

Adults

- Genetic factors
- Physical inactivity/sedentary behaviors
- Diet
- Socioeconomic factors
- Medications
- Medical conditions
- Gut bacteria

Children/adolescents

- Physical inactivity/lack of sports participation
- Diet
- Sugar-sweetened beverages
- Television viewing
- Electronic games

Individuals with the highest genetic risk had BMIs that were only 2.7 kg/m^2 higher than those with a low genetic risk.[18]

Physical Activity

Physical activity provides the largest contribution to significant energy expenditure. The American College of Sports Medicine recommends that 150 to 250 minutes of moderate intensity exercise per week is needed to prevent weight gain when accompanied by appropriate dietary interventions.[19] However, appropriate levels of physical activity to prevent weight gain are not required in modern daily activities of daily living for most people.[20] Life in most developed (and some developing) nations does not require the same levels of activity for subsistence that was required in the past.[20] Technology has made it easier to be productive while being mostly sedentary.[20] As an example, television viewing has a clear and significant association with obesity.[21] Even after adjusting for age, smoking, exercise level, and dietary factors, every 2-hour increment spent watching TV is associated with a 23% increase in obesity.[21] In the context of modern living, sufficient physical activity is a cornerstone of weight management. However, according to the Surgeon General's report on physical activity, the percentage of adults living in the United States who participate in physical activity continues to decline with age.[22]

Caloric Intake

The global food supply has changed significantly over the last half-century. The availability of cheap, convenient, calorically dense food has contributed significantly to the increase in obesity.[23] Specifically, an increase in carbohydrate and fat content in foods processed outside the home has been linked to obesity.[24] The increase in body weight during middle age is particularly associated with increased intake of potato chips, sugar-sweetened beverages, unprocessed red meats, and processed meats.[24] Body weight is inversely associated with a diet high in fruits, vegetables, whole grains, nuts, and yogurt.[24] The intake of sugar-sweetened beverages is also increasingly implicated in excess weight gain.[25] Highlighting the complex interplay between genetic and environmental factors, there seems to be a genetic predisposition for excess weight gain associated with the intake of sugar-sweetened beverages.[26]

Socioeconomic Status

Socioeconomic status is another well-established risk factor associated with overweight and obesity. The role socioeconomic status plays in the obesity pandemic has shifted over the past century. In the mid–twentieth century, obesity in the United States and Europe was directly associated with income. Individuals with more income were more likely to be overweight or obese.[27] That relationship no longer holds. Obesity is more prevalent in lower socioeconomic groups.[28,29] The relationship between wealth and obesity is multifactorial and likely related to factors such as nutrition, neighborhood food environments, education, and the built environment (the safety of people's neighborhood, access to playgrounds and sidewalks, transportation, number of fast food restaurants, neighborhood trails, and social services).[30,31]

Miscellaneous Risk Factors

A variety of other factors place people at risk of becoming obese or overweight. Certain medications (eg, glucocorticoids, antidiabetic medications, antidepressants, and antipsychotics) increase risk for weight gain. Certain disease states (eg, Cushing syndrome, hypothyroidism, and polycystic ovary syndrome) are associated with excess weight gain. An individual's microbiome has also been shown to play a role in energy metabolism and risk of obesity.[32]

Risk in Children and Adolescents

As with adults, environmental factors, such as caloric intake and lack of physical activity, play a significant role in the development of obesity in children and adolescents. Sugar-sweetened beverage intake contributes to obesity as well.[25,33] Excess screen time is associated with higher BMI in children.[34] The excess use of electronic games is related to obesity in childhood.[35] The association between obesity and television watching is stronger than that between obesity and electronic games in children, likely because gaming requires some degree of emotional or physical participation.[34] Advertising energy-dense foods specifically to children is also more prevalent on television.[34] Participation in sports is inversely related to overweight/obesity in children and adolescents.[36,37] The reduction in school sports programs has likely contributed to an increase in the rates of obese and overweight children and adolescents.[36]

PREVALENCE/INCIDENCE IN THE UNITED STATES

The prevalence of overweight and obesity in the United States is has important implications. The prevalence of overweight and obesity in the United States has increased to the point at which people who are overweight or obese outnumber normal-weight individuals by 2:1. In addition, the prevalence of severe obesity has increased to 7%.[7] Nearly 85% of American adults will be either overweight or obese by the year 2030.[6] Obesity rates increased from 24% in 1990 to 37% in 2010 for individuals more than 60 years of age.[38] Obesity rates in Hispanic people and non-Hispanic black people were 43% and 48% respectively in 2012.[8] Compared with men, women are disproportionately affected by severe obesity regardless of age or race.[8] However, rates of obesity seem to have plateaued at 35% between 2003 to 2004 and 2011 to 2012.[8]

Equally serious, overweight and obesity rates in children parallel those of adults. Nearly one-third of American children are either overweight or obese.[8] The prevalence of obesity in children between 2011 and 2012 was 17%.[8] This percentage also seems to have stabilized, because obesity rates in children did not change significantly between 2004 and 2010.[8] As with adults, although rates of obesity in children seem to have stabilized, the prevalence of severe obesity has continued to increase. From the period 1976 to 1980 through 2012, the rate of severe obesity in children increased from 1% to 6%.[39]

WORLDWIDE/REGIONAL INCIDENCE

Worldwide, the prevalence of overweight and obesity increased by 28% for adults from 1980 to 2013[4] (**Fig. 1**). From 1980 to 2013, the number of overweight and obese people increased from 857 million to 2.1 billion. Worldwide, 37% of men and 38% of women are estimated to have a BMI greater than 25 kg/m^2.[4,23] At present, 50% of obese individuals live in only 10 countries (United States, China, India, Russia, Brazil, Mexico, Egypt, Germany, Pakistan, and Indonesia). In Europe, 17% of adults are obese and current trends place Europe on an obesity trajectory similar to the United States.[40] Significant regional variations exist in Europe as well, suggesting that socioeconomic conditions play a role in the development of obesity.[41] Specifically, 20% of men and 22% of women in Belgium are obese, and 25% of men and women in the United Kingdom are obese. In other areas of the world, 21% of men and 33% of

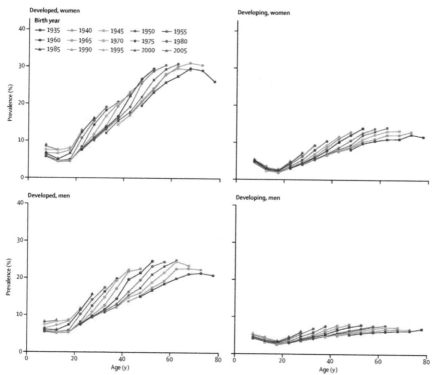

Fig. 1. Prevalence of obesity by age across birth cohorts for men and women in developed and developing countries. (*From* Ng M, Fleming T, Robinson M, et al. Global, regional, and national prevalence of overweight and obesity in children and adults during 1980–2013: a systematic analysis for the Global Burden of Disease Study 2013. Lancet 2014;384(9945):770; with permission.)

women in Mexico are obese, 14% of men and women in Pakistan are obese, 11% of men and 10% of women in China are obese, and 13.5% of men and 42% of women in South Africa are obese.[4,42]

Rates of obesity are increasing in developing countries as well.[4] Although age-adjusted rates of obesity are lower in developing compared with developed countries, 62% of the world's obese people live in developing countries.[4] The WHO suggest that, as undernourished populations decline,[43] obesity becomes more important as a public health disease in low-income countries. Sub-Saharan Africa is the only region of the world in which obesity is not common.[44] In the developing world, rates of overweight and obesity seem higher in women than in men.[4]

Overweight and obesity are also increasing in children and adolescents around the globe. From 1980 to 2013, the prevalence of overweight and obesity in children and adolescents in developed countries increased from 17% to 24% in boys and from 16% to 23% in girls.[4] During the same time period, the prevalence of overweight and obesity increased from 8% to 13% in boys and from 8% to 13% in girls in developing countries.[4] Direct comparisons between countries are more difficult in children and adolescents than in adults because of different classification systems of overweight and obesity. Despite this, in countries with comparable statistics, rates of overweight and obesity in children and adolescents exceed 30% in Greece, Italy, Great

Britain, Spain, and Portugal.[45] Thirteen percent of children and adolescents are over-weight or obese in China. Fifteen percent of Israeli boys, 12% of boys in Chile, 11% of boys in Mexico, 18% of girls in Uruguay, and 12% of girls in Costa Rica are also re-ported to be overweight or obese.[4,46]

MORBIDITY AND MORTALITY

Obesity is an independent risk factor for excess morbidity and mortality. Although exact numbers are difficult to define, in 2000, 15% of deaths in the United States were attributable to excess weight.[47] Obesity contributes to an estimated 111,909 to 365,000 deaths in the United States and at least 2.8 million deaths worldwide each year.[48,49] Globally, overweight and obesity are estimated to be the fifth leading cause of death.[49] People with a greater BMI have a greater risk of all-cause mortal-ity.[50] For both women and men, obesity as an adult is associated with a significant reduction in life expectancy. Compared with normal-weight individuals, obese pa-tients have a higher all-cause mortality.[7,51] Data from the Framingham Study indi-cate that people who were obese at age 40 years died 6 to 7 years earlier than normal-weight peers.[52] Individuals who are overweight at age 40 years have a life expectancy that is 3 years less their normal-weight peers.[52] The life expectancy in severely obese individuals is even worse. Median survival is decreased 8 to 10 years in this group.[50] Data from the Prospective Studies Collaboration analysis showed that overall mortality was lowest at a BMI of 22.5 to 25 kg/m^2.[50] Every 5 kg/m^2 increase in BMI was associated with a 30% increase in all-cause mortality[50] (Fig. 2).

In addition to the increased risk of overall mortality, overweight and obesity are associated with an increased risk for multiple morbidities.[27] The risk of developing a chronic disease (hypertension, heart disease, gallstones, colon cancer, and stroke) increases with increasing BMI.[53,54] One of the strongest associations is with diabetes mellitus. More than 80% of type 2 diabetes is attributable to over-weight and obesity.[55] Overweight individuals have a 3-fold higher risk and obese in-dividuals have a 7-fold higher risk of developing type 2 diabetes compared with normal-weight individuals.[56] The American Diabetes Association (ADA) recom-mends any patient more than 45 years of age who is overweight or obese be tested for type 2 diabetes even if they are asymptomatic.[57] The ADA also recommends that patients who are severely obese be tested for type 2 diabetes regardless of age.[57] Individuals who are metabolically healthy (no history of insulin resistance, poor glycemic control, hypertension, or dyslipidemia) but are obese have a 4-fold higher risk of developing type 2 diabetes than those who are metabolically healthy and of normal weight.[58]

In addition to BMI, the distribution of body fat influences the risk of developing type 2 diabetes. NHANES III showed that individuals with high waist circumference values (men, >102 cm [40 inches]; and women, >89 cm [35 inches]) were more likely to develop diabetes, hypertension, and dyslipidemia than those with a normal waist circumference.[59] Obesity is associated with hyperinsulinism and insulin resistance (before the onset of overt hyperglycemia). Individuals who lose weight decrease their risk for type 2 diabetes.[60]

Obesity also increases the risk of certain cancers in both men and women. In 2007, 6% of all cancers were associated with obesity.[61] A 5 kg/m^2 increase in BMI in men is associated with an increased risk of renal, colon, thyroid, and esophageal cancers.[62] A 5 kg/m^2 increase in BMI for women was associated with an increased risk of endome-trial, renal, esophageal, and gallbladder cancer.[62]

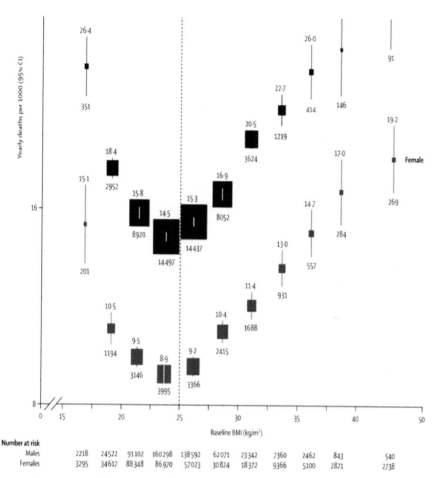

Fig. 2. All-cause mortality versus BMI for each sex in the range 15 to 50 kg/m² (excluding the first 5 years of follow-up). Relative risk at ages 35 to 89 years, adjusted for age at risk, smoking, and study, were multiplied by a common factor (ie, floated) to make the weighted average match the prospective studies collaboration (PSC) mortality at ages 35 to 79 years. Floated mortalities are shown above each square and numbers of deaths below. Area of square is inversely proportional to the variance of the log risk. Boundaries of BMI groups are indicated by tick marks. Ninety-five percent confidence intervals (CIs) for the floated rates reflect uncertainty in the log risk for each single rate. Dotted vertical line indicates 25 kg/m² (boundary between upper and lower BMI ranges in this report). (*From* Prospective Studies Collaboration. Body-mass index and cause-specific mortality in 900 000 adults: collaborative analyses of 57 prospective studies. Lancet 2009;373(9669):1087; with permission.)

Obesity has a particularly strong relationship with cardiovascular disease. Obesity is associated with an increase in the risk of stroke, heart failure, atrial fibrillation, lipid abnormalities, coronary disease, and hypertension. Along with ischemic heart disease, stroke is one of the leading causes of death around the world.[63] Multiple studies show an increased risk of ischemic stroke with increasing BMI.[64–66] In the Framingham Heart Study, obesity was thought to be causal in 14% of cases of heart failure for women and 11% of cases of heart failure for men.[67] Obesity also increases the risk of developing atrial fibrillation.[68] Lipid abnormalities, including a reduction in high-density lipoprotein cholesterol along with an increase in low-density lipoprotein cholesterol, very-low-density lipoprotein cholesterol, triglycerides, and total cholesterol, are associated with obesity.[69] Coronary heart disease is significantly increased in both overweight and obese individuals.[70] Overweight and obesity account for nearly 26% of hypertension in men and 28% of hypertension in women.[71] There is a 2-fold or higher risk of developing hypertension, coronary heart disease, and stroke in children who are obese.[72]

Compared with normal-weight individuals, obese individuals have a 30% greater chance of mortality from surgery and a 50% increase in the risk of major complications from surgery.[27] Obesity is associated with a 45% increased risk of overall mortality, higher rates of complications, and longer time in the intensive care unit in patients with trauma.[73] Obese individuals are at increased risk of surgical site, intensive care unit, urinary tract, and other infections during hospitalizations. Obese individuals are also at higher risk of acquiring respiratory tract infections during influenza season.[74,75]

Osteoarthritis risk increases with increasing BMI as well. Obesity is second only to age as the predominant risk factor for osteoarthritis.[76] Excess mechanical forces lead to excessive joint loading and early osteoarthritis of the knee in obese individuals.[77] Osteoarthritis of non–weight-bearing joints such as the hand and wrist also occurs at higher rates in obese patients.[78,79] However, rates of osteoarthritis decrease in patients who lose weight.[80]

COSTS OF OBESITY

Calculating the exact cost of obesity is difficult. Estimates for the costs of obesity in the United States range from $147 billion to $210 billion per year,[9] which represents roughly 21% of annual United States health care expenditures.[9] Per capita spending on health care is $2741 higher per person for obese individuals.[9] Compared with normal-weight people, obese individuals are responsible for 46% higher inpatient costs, 27% more outpatient visits, and 80% higher spending on prescription medications.[10] Obesity-related medical costs are projected to increase sharply over the next decade in the United States.[81]

More than $14 billion in direct costs are associated with the treatment of obesity in children and adolescents.[82] Medicaid data suggest that obese children account for $6730 annually in health care costs compared with $2446 in health care costs for normal-weight children.[83] Hospitalizations of children with obesity between 1999 and 2005 almost doubled, whereas total health care costs of obesity-related hospitalizations increased to nearly $238 million in 2005.[84]

SUMMARY

Obesity is a worldwide epidemic associated with increased morbidity and mortality and a significant burden to health care systems worldwide. Obesity is a complex disease affecting large numbers of people throughout the world. A complex combination of genetic, environmental, and social factors in an increasingly technical world with increased availability of cheap, calorically dense foods has created the perfect conditions for sharp increases in rates of overweight and obesity across the globe.

REFERENCES

1. Hu FB. Obesity epidemiology. Oxford (Untied Kingdom): Oxford University Press; 2008. p. 498.

2. National Institute of Health, National Heart, Lung, and Blood Institute. Clinical guidelines on the identification, evaluation, and treatment of overweight and obesity in adults: the evidence report. Obes Res 1998;6(Suppl 2):515.
3. Ogden CL, Flegal KM. Changes in terminology for childhood overweight and obesity. Natl Health Stat Report 2010;25:1–5.
4. NG M, Fleming T, Robinson M, et al. Global, regional, and national prevalence of overweight and obesity in children and adults during 1980-2013: a systematic analysis for the Global Burden of Disease Study 2013. Lancet 2014;384:766–81.
5. Kelly T, Yang W, Chen C-S, et al. Global burden of obesity in 2005 and projections in 2030. Int J Obes 2008;32(9):1431–7.
6. Wang Y, Beydoun MA, Liang L, et al. Will all Americans become overweight or obese? Estimating the progression and cost of the US obesity epidemic. Obesity (Silver Spring) 2008;16(10):2323–30.
7. Flegal KM, Kit BK, Orpana H, et al. Association of all-cause mortality with overweight and obesity using standard body mass index categories: a systematic review and meta-analysis. JAMA 2013;309:71.
8. Ogden CL, Carrol MD, Kit BK, et al. Prevalence of childhood and adult obesity in the United States, 2011-2012. JAMA 2014;311:806.
9. Cawley J, Meyerhoefer C. The medical care cost of obesity: an instrumental variables approach. J Health Econ 2012;31(1):219–30.
10. Finkelstein EA, Trogdon JG, Coehn JW, et al. Annual medical spending attributable to obesity: payer and service specific estimates. Heath Aff (Millwood) 2009;28:822–31.
11. WHO Consultation on Obesity. Obesity: preventing and managing the global epidemic. Geneva, 3–5 June 1997. Geneva (Switzerland): World Health Organization; 1998.
12. Jensen MD, Ryan DH, Apovian CM, et al. 2013 AHA/ACC/TOS guideline for the management of overweight and obesity in adults: a report of the American College of Cardiology/American Heart Association Task Force on Practice Guidelines and The Obesity Society. Circulation 2014;129:S102.
13. WHO Expert Consultation. Appropriate body mass index for Asian populations and its implications for policy and intervention strategies. Lancet 2004;363:157.
14. Grummer-Strawn LM, Reinold C, Krebs NF, Centers for Disease Control and Prevention (CDC). Use of World Health Organization and CDC growth charts for children aged 0-59 months in the United States. MMWR Recomm Rep 2010;59(rr-9):1–15.
15. Peters JC, Wyatt HR, Donahoo WT, et al. From instinct to intellect: the challenge of maintaining healthy weight in the modern world. Obes Rev 2002;3:69–74.
16. Wardle J, Carnell S, Haworth CM, et al. Evidence for a strong genetic influence on childhood adiposity despite the force of the obesogenic environment. Am J Clin Nutr 2008;87:398.
17. Peruse L, Rankinen T, Zuberi A, et al. The human obesity gene map: the 2004 update. Obes Res 2005;13:381.
18. Speliiotes EK, Willer CJ, Berndt SI, et al. Association analyses of 249,796 individuals reveal 18 new loci associated with body mass index. Nat Genet 2010;42(11):937–48.
19. Donnelly JE, Blair SN, Jakicic JM, et al. American College of Sports Medicine Position Stand. Appropriate physical activity intervention strategies for weight loss and prevention of weight regain for adults. Med Sci Sports Exerc 2009;41(2):459–71.
20. Mitchell N, Catenacci V, Wyatt H, et al. Obesity: overview of an epidemic. Psychiatr Clin North Am 2011;34(3):717–32.

21. Hu FB, Li TY, Colditz GA, et al. Television watching and other sedentary behaviors in relation to risk of obesity and type 2 diabetes mellitus in women. JAMA 2003; 289:1785.

22. US Department of Health and Human Services. Physical activity and health: a report of the Surgeon General. Atlanta (GA): US Department of Health and Human Services, Centers for Disease Control and Prevention, National Center for Chronic Disease Prevention and Health Promotion; 1996.

23. Swinburn BA, Sacks G, Hall KD, et al. The global obesity pandemic: shaped by global drivers and local environments. Lancet 2011;378:804.

24. Mozaffarian D, Hao T, Rimm EB, et al. Changes in diet and lifestyle and long-term weight gain in women and men. N Engl J Med 2011;364:2392.

25. Malik VS, Pan A, Willett WC, et al. Sugar-sweetened beverages and weight gain in children and adults: a systematic review and meta-analysis. Am J Clin Nutr 2013;98:1084.

26. Qi Q, Chu AY, Kang JH, et al. Sugar sweetened beverages and genetic risk of obesity. N Engl J Med 2012;367:1387.

27. Hruby A, Hu FB. The epidemiology of obesity: a big picture. Pharmacoeconomics 2014;33(7):673–89.

28. Drewnowski A, Rehm CD, Solet D. Disparities in obesity rates: analysis by ZIP code area. Soc Sci Med 2007;65:2458.

29. Koh KA, Hoy JS, O'Connell JJ, et al. The hunger-obesity paradox: obesity in the homeless. J Urban Health 2012;89(6):952–64.

30. Drewnowski A. The economics of food choice behavior: why poverty and obesity are linked. Nestle Nutr Inst Workshop Ser 2012;73:95.

31. Dubowitz T, Ghosh-Dastidar MB, Steiner E, et al. Are our actions aligned with our evidence? The skinny on changing the landscape of obesity. Obesity (Silver Spring) 2013;21:419.

32. Clarke SF, Murphy EF, Nilaweera K, et al. The gut microbiota and its relationship to diet and obesity: new insights. Gut Microbes 2012;3(3):186–202.

33. DeBoer MD, Scharf RJ, Demmer RT. Sugar-sweetened beverages and weight gain in 2- to 5-year-old children. Pediatrics 2013;132:413.

34. Bickham DS, Blood EA, Walls CE, et al. Characteristics of screen media use associated with higher BMI in young adolescents. Pediatrics 2013;131(935): 935–41.

35. Stettler N, Signer TM, Suter PM. Electronic games and environmental factors associated with childhood obesity in Switzerland. Obes Res 2004;12:896.

36. Drake KM, Beach ML, Longacre MR, et al. Influence of sports, physical education, and active commuting to school on adolescent weight status. Pediatrics 2012; 130(2):e296–305.

37. Flegal KM, Carroll MD, Kit BK, et al. Prevalence of obesity and trends in the distribution of body mass index among US adults 1999-2010. JAMA 2012;307:491.

38. Mathus-Vliegen EMH, Basdevant A, Finer N, et al. Prevalence, pathophysiology, health consequences and treatment options of obesity in the elderly: a guideline. Obes Facts 2012;5:460–83.

39. Skinner AC, Skelton JA. Prevalence and trends in obesity and severe obesity among children in the United States, 1999-2012. JAMA Pediatr 2014;168:561.

40. Von Ruesten A, Steffen A, Floegel A, et al. Trend in obesity prevalence in European adult cohort populations during follow-up since 1996 and their predictions to 2015. PLoS One 2011;6(11):E27455.

41. Berghofer A, Pischon T, Reinhold T, et al. Obesity prevalence from a European perspective: a systematic review. BMC Public Health 2008;8(1):200.

42. International Association for the Study of Obesity. Available at: http://www.iaso. org/resources/world-map-obesity. Accessed September 1, 2015.
43. Sattar N, McConnachie A, Shaper AG, et al. Can metabolic syndrome usefully predict cardiovascular disease and diabetes? Outcome data from two prospective studies. Lancet 2008;371:1927–35.
44. Haslam WD, James WP. Obesity. Lancet 2005;366:1197–209.
45. Janssen I, Katzmarzyk PT, Boyce WF, et al. Comparison of overweight and obesity prevalence in school-aged youth from 34 countries and their relationships with physical activity and dietary patterns. Obes Rev 2005;6:123.
46. Liang Y-J, Xi B, Song A-Q, et al. Trends in general abdominal obesity among Chinese children and adolescents 1993-2009: general and abdominal obesity in Chinese children. Pediatr Obes 2012;7(5):355–64.
47. Mokdad AH, Marks JS, Stroup DF, et al. Actual causes of death in the United States, 2000. JAMA 2004;291(10):1238–45.
48. Flegal KM, Graubard BI, Williamson DF, et al. Excess deaths associated with underweight, overweight, and obesity. JAMA 2005;293:1861.
49. Ellulu M, Abed Y, Rahmat A, et al. Epidemiology of obesity in developing countries: challenges and prevention. Glo Epidemi Obes 2014;2:2.
50. Prospective Studies Collaboration, Whitlock G, Lewington S, Sherliker P, et al. Body-mass index and cause-specific mortality in 900,000 adults: collaborative analyses of 57 prospective studies. Lancet 2009;373:1083.
51. McTigue K, Larson JC, Valoski A, et al. Mortality and cardiac and vascular outcomes in extremely obese women. JAMA 2006;296:79.
52. Peeters A, Barendregt JJ, Willekens F, et al. Obesity in adulthood and its consequences for life expectancy: a life-table analysis. Ann Intern Med 2003;138(1): 24–32.
53. Field AE, Coakley EH, Must A, et al. Impact of overweight on the risk of developing common chronic diseases during a 10 year period. Arch Intern Med 2001;161: 1581.
54. Willett WC, Dietz WH, Colditz GA. Guidelines for healthy weight. N Engl J Med 1999;341:427.
55. National Diabetes Information Clearinghouse, US Department of Health and Human Services. Diabetes fact sheet. Available at: http://diabetes.niddk.nih.gov/dm/pubs/ overview/. Accessed September 1, 2015.
56. Abdullah A, Peeters A, de Courten M, et al. The magnitude of association between overweight and obesity and the risk of diabetes: a meta-analysis of prospective cohort studies. Diabetes Res Clin Pract 2010;89(3):309–19.
57. American Diabetes Association. Standards of medical care in diabetes – 2012. Diabetes Care 2012;35(Suppl 1):S11–63.
58. Bell JA, Kivimaki M, Hamer M. Metabolically healthy obesity and risk of incident type 2 diabetes: a meta-analysis of prospective cohort studies. Obes Rev 2014; 15(6):504–15.
59. Janssen I, Katzmarzk PT, Ross R. Body mass index, waist circumference, and health risk: evidence in support of current National Institutes of Health guidelines. Arch Intern Med 2002;162:2074.
60. Knowler WC, Barrett-Connor E, Fowler SE, et al. Reduction in the incidence of type 2 diabetes with lifestyle intervention or metformin. N Engl J Med 2002; 346:393.
61. Polednak AP. Estimating the number of U.S. incident cancers attributable to obesity and the impact on temporal trends in incidence rates for obesity-related cancers. Cancer Detect Prev 2008;32(3):190–9.

62. Renehan AG, Tyson M, Egger M, et al. Body-mass index and incidence of cancer: a systematic review and meta-analysis of prospective observational studies. Lancet 2008;371:569.

63. Lozano R, Naghavi M, Foreman K, et al. Global and regional mortality from 235 causes of death for 20 age groups in 1990 and 2010: a systematic analysis for the Global Burden of Disease Study 2010. Lancet 2012;380(9859):2095–128.

64. Emerging Risk Factors Collaboration, Wormser D, Kaptoge S, Di Angelantonio E, et al. Separate and combined associations of body-mass index and abdominal adiposity with cardiovascular disease: collaborative analysis of 58 prospective studies. Lancet 2011;377:1085.

65. Kurth T, Gaziano JM, Rexrode KM, et al. Prospective study of body mass index and risk of stroke in apparently health women. Circulation 2005;111:1992.

66. Kurth T, Gaziano JM, Berger K, et al. Body mass index and the risk of stroke in men. Arch Intern Med 2002;162:2557.

67. Kenchaiah S, Evans JC, Levy D, et al. Obesity and the risk of heart failure. N Engl J Med 2002;347:305.

68. Wang TJ, Parise H, Levy D, et al. Obesity and the risk of new-onset atrial fibrillation. JAMA 2004;292:2471.

69. Poirier P, Giles TD, Bray GA, et al. Obesity and cardiovascular disease: pathophysiology, evaluation, and effect of weight loss. Arterioscler Thromb Vasc Biol 2006;26:968.

70. Global Burden of Metabolic Risk Factors for Chronic Diseases Collaboration (BMI Mediated Effects), Lu Y, Hajifathalian K, Ezzati M, et al. Metabolic mediators of the effects of body-mass index, overweight, obesity on coronary heart disease and stroke: a pooled analysis of 97 prospective cohorts with 1.8 million participants. Lancet 2014;383:970.

71. Wilson PW, D'Agostino RB, Sullivan L, et al. Overweight and obesity as determinants of cardiovascular risk: the Framingham experience. Arch Intern Med 2002; 162:1867.

72. Reilly JJ, Kelly J. Long-term impact of overweight and obesity in childhood and adolescence on morbidity and premature mortality in adulthood: systematic review. Int J Obes 2011;35(7):891–8.

73. Liu T, Chen J, Bai X, et al. The effect of obesity on outcomes in trauma patients: a meta-analysis. Injury 2013;44(9):1145–52.

74. Huttunen R, Syrjanen J. Obesity and the risk and outcome of infection. Int J Obes 2013;37(3):333–40.

75. Almond MH, Edwards MR, Barclay WS, et al. Obesity and susceptibility to severe outcomes following respiratory viral infection. Thorax 2013;68:684.

76. Radin EL, Paul IL, Rose PM. Role of mechanical factors in pathogenesis of primary osteoarthritis. Lancet 1972;1:519–22.

77. Felson DT, Anderson JJ, Naimark A, et al. Obesity and knee osteoarthritis. The Framingham Study. Ann Intern Med 1988;109:179–89.

78. Grotle M, Hagen KB, Natvig B, et al. Obesity and osteoarthritis in knee, hip, and/or hand: an epidemiological study in the general population with 10 years follow-up. BMC Musculoskelet Disord 2008;9:132.

79. Carman WJ, Sowers M, Hawthorne VM, et al. Obesity as a risk factor for osteoarthritis of the hand and wrist: a prospective study. Am J Epidemiol 1994;139: 119–29.

80. Felson DT, Zhang Y, Anthony JM, et al. Weight loss reduces the risk for symptomatic knee osteoarthritis in women. The Framingham Study. Ann Intern Med 1992; 116:535.

81. Wang CY, McPherson K, Marsh T, et al. Health and economic burden of the projected obesity trends in the USA and the UK. Lancet 2011;378:815–25.

82. Trasande L, Chatterjee S. The impact of obesity on health service utilization and costs in childhood. Obesity 2009;17(9):1749–54.

83. Marder W, Chang S. Childhood obesity, costs, treatment patterns, disparities in care, and prevalent medical conditions. Thomson Medstat Res Brief. Ann Arbor (MI): Thompson Medstat; 2006.

84. Trasande L, Liu Y, Fryer G, et al. Effects of childhood obesity on hospital care and costs, 1999-2005. Health Aff 2009;23(4):751–60.

Obesity in Older Adults

Virginia B. Kalish, MD

KEYWORDS

- Obesity • Elderly • Older adults • Mortality • Physical function • Weight loss

KEY POINTS

- Older overweight and obese adults do not have the same risk of morbidity and mortality as younger patients, particularly if obesity develops late in life.
- Compared with young and middle-aged individuals, body mass indices (BMIs) in the obese range are associated with a relative decrease in the risk for all-cause mortality in adults aged 65 to 74 years. There is not enough evidence to make an association in persons 75 years of age or older.
- Higher BMI imparts an increased risk for diabetes, osteoarthritis, and disability, and a protective effect on bone density and hip fracture in older adults.
- Weight management plans should be individualized for obese elderly patients. A critical goal is to maintain or increase quality of life and physical function.
- Weight loss, intentional or unintentional, is accompanied by a decline in fat free mass. Therefore, activities to maintain muscle strength, such as progressive resistance training, should be a component of all weight loss plans for the elderly.

INTRODUCTION

The world is aging as obesity is rising. By the year 2030, over-65 year olds will make up 20% of the US population. By 2035, 25% of Europe's populace will be 65 or older.[1] Concurrently, adult obesity prevalence has steadily climbed in the United States since 1976 to 1980.[2] Worldwide, overweight and obesity have overtaken malnutrition in terms of overall health risk.[3] Accordingly, the prevalence of obesity is increasing in most developed and rapidly developing nations[1,4–7] (**Table 1**). The convergence of aging and obesity will likely carry significant financial and societal burdens.[6,7] Less is known about the benefits and risks of obesity in elderly patients compared with children and adults. Management strategies for obese elderly patients differ from children and adults as well.[6,8]

BODY COMPOSITION CHANGES WITH AGE

Total body fat increases with age and peaks at 70.[4] There is an associated redistribution of fat from subcutaneous regions to intra-abdominal, intrahepatic, and intramuscular

Department of Family Medicine, National Capital Consortium Family Medicine Residency, Fort Belvoir Community Hospital, 9300 Dewitt Loop, Fort Belvoir, VA 22060, USA
E-mail address: virginia.b.kalish.civ@mail.mil

Prim Care Clin Office Pract 43 (2016) 137–144
http://dx.doi.org/10.1016/j.pop.2015.10.002
0095-4543/16/$ – see front matter Published by Elsevier Inc.
primarycare.theclinics.com

Table 1			
Percentage of overweight and obese older adults in the US population			
BMI	Age (y)	Male (%)	Female (%)
≥25	65–74	76.9	73.8
	≥75	70.4	62.4
≥30	65–74	36.4	44.2
	≥75	27.4	29.8

Data from U.S. Department of Health and Human Services. Health, United States, 2014: with special feature on adults aged 55–64. 2015. Available at: http://www.cdc.gov/nchs/data/hus/hus14.pdf#064. Accessed June 12, 2015.

regions. Sarcopenic obesity describes the combination of age-related muscle atrophy and increase in adiposity. A decrease in total energy expenditure coupled with normal hormonal changes accounts for increases in total body fat. Basal metabolic rate, physical activity, and muscle strength decrease with age. Testosterone and growth hormone production decline, as does the responsiveness to thyroid hormone and leptin.[4,5,9–10]

BODY MASS INDEX AS A MEASURE FOR OBESITY AND A PROGNOSTIC INDICATOR

- At the same body mass index (BMI), older adults have a greater proportion of body fat compared with younger adults.
- There is no consensus regarding the best measure of obesity in the older population.
- In the elderly, the prognostic importance of BMI is not clear.

BMI is a common screening tool used to define overweight and obesity. In 1998, the National Heart, Lung, and Blood Institute (NHLBI) defined overweight and obese persons, regardless of age, as a BMI of 25 to 29.9 kg/m² and greater than or equal to 30 kg/m², respectively.[11] The obesity cutoff (30 kg/m²) was derived from a correlation with increased all-cause mortality. BMI is an easy screening tool that correlates with percentage body fat in young and middle-aged adults. With aging, however, normal changes in body composition render BMI less accurate.[5,7,10,11] As fat mass increases and lean mass decreases, BMI underestimates total adiposity. Most elderly patients also decline in height, resulting in an overall overestimation of obesity.

Updated National Institutes of Health/NHLBI guidelines[2] use the combination of BMI and waist circumference (WC) as a prognostic indicator. Waist-to-hip ratio is associated with geriatric mortality.[12] WC combined with midarm muscle circumference is an effective measure of lean body mass and correlates inversely with all-cause mortality.[4] Unfortunately, no consensus has yet emerged regarding a superior alternative measurement to BMI in the elderly. Further research is needed to identify levels associated with risk.

THE RELATIONSHIP BETWEEN BODY MASS INDEX AND MORTALITY

- Unlike younger individuals, overweight elderly patients do not carry an elevated risk for all-cause or cardiovascular mortality (**Table 2**). For obese patients aged 60 to 75 years, there is an inverse relationship between relative mortality risk and BMI.
- A consistent association between cardiovascular and all-cause mortality and BMI has not been demonstrated in persons greater than 75 years of age.

Table 2
Body mass index as a prognostic indicator for all-cause and cardiovascular mortality in older adults

Age	Association Between BMI and All-Cause Mortality	Optimal BMI Range (All-Cause and Cardiovascular Mortality)
65–74	Wide-based U-shaped curve,[13,14] decreased or neutral[4]	27–30,[13,14] 25–35[4]
>75	No association[9]	Unknown

Data from Refs.[4,13,14]

Whereas obesity is associated with an increased mortality risk in young and middle-aged persons, a similar relationship is not seen for adults aged 60 to 75 years; this has been called the "obesity survival paradox."[4] An alternative interpretation is based on the U-shaped curve phenomenon. If BMI is plotted against mortality, a BMI of less than or equal to 18.5 to 23.5 kg/m^2 and greater than or equal to 27 to 32 kg/m^2 imparts an increase in all-cause mortality in older adults 65 to 74 years of age.[13,14] The right arm of the U has a gentle incline, indicating a progressive increase in BMI is associated with minimal excess mortality risk.[13] Optimal BMI increases with increasing age.[13] This relationship diminishes and then ceases as one reaches 75 years of age or older.[13] There is conflicting evidence for an association with BMI and cardiovascular mortality in persons less than 75, and when an association has been found, it is not strong.[13] Underweight elderly may have unintentional weight loss, higher risk for malnutrition, osteoporosis, falls, and hip fracture, explaining the left arm of the U-shaped curve.[4,13]

POTENTIAL EXPLANATIONS FOR IMPROVED SURVIVABILITY IN THE OBESE ELDER

- BMI does not accurately measure percentage body fat in older adults.
- There may be a selective survival bias, in which the metabolically healthy obese (MHO) are overrepresented as they outlive the metabolically unhealthy obese (MUHO).
- Weight gain that occurs in old age decreases the time to develop obesity-related complications.
- Unintentional weight loss may confound many observational studies, thereby skewing the relative mortality risk in favor of the overweight and obese.

The relationship between BMI and mortality in the elderly comes from observational data, preventing any conclusions regarding causality. Multiple factors contribute to the notion that older obese adults have improved survivability, including the failure of the BMI measure to accurately reflect changes in total body fat with aging. Adiposity may also impart some degree of protection, as seen in other disease states, such as cancer, HIV, heart failure, and hemodialysis.[4,10] In addition, overweight and obese elderly have outlived their counterparts and may have a survival advantage due to a healthier phenotype.[1,15] Such individuals are referred to as MHO.[12] MHO individuals have increased BMI, but less abdominal fat deposition and a smaller WC than MUHO individuals.[12] MHO have greater insulin sensitivity, fewer inflammatory markers, and favorable hormonal and immune profiles.[16] Cardiovascular risk factors, such as elevated low-density lipoprotein and blood pressure, may not carry the same degree of risk in MHO elderly as compared with younger individuals.[13] Study designs that control for obesity-related pre-existing disease may overrepresent the MHO population among the survivors, further diminishing the overall magnitude of obesity risk.[13]

Studies suggest that although excess midlife adiposity increases mortality risk, weight gain at age 70 does not.[4] When weight gain occurs in late life, there is less time to impose metabolic and cardiovascular health risks.[9,13] Unintentional weight loss in late life, on the other hand, increases relative mortality risk.[4,13]

BODY MASS INDEX AND MORBIDITY IN OLDER ADULTS

- Overweight older adults are at increased risk for osteoarthritis, diabetes, and disability but otherwise do not carry the same risk for morbidity as overweight young and middle-aged individuals (**Table 3**).
- When BMI increases into the obesity range in older adults, an association with cardiovascular morbidity and some cancers begins to appear. Obese elders have higher rates of functional disability and a greater risk for institutionalization.
- Obesity protects against bone density loss and hip fracture.

Most studies describing obesity-related complications have been performed in younger populations.[10,11] Obesity and aging are independent risk factors for multiple conditions. In older adults, a BMI greater than or equal to 25 kg/m^2 is associated with diabetes, osteoarthritis, and physical disability. A BMI in the overweight range does not, however, confer an increased risk for cardiovascular disease (CVD), urinary incontinence, sleep apnea, and cancer.[19] As BMI creeps into the obese range, risk for some cancers and CVD increases,[17] but rates of CVD mortality do not. Visceral adiposity is independently associated with metabolic syndrome in adults aged 70 to 79 years,[10,11] and yet metabolic syndrome does not have the same prognostic value in older persons as it does in the young and middle aged.[20] Obesity and aging, both conditions of chronic inflammation, result in disability, mobility impairment, decreased quality of life,[2] increased costs, and institutionalization.[10,11,14,21,22] An

Table 3 Obesity as a risk factor for morbidity	
Outcome	**Obesity Risk Association**
Cancers (breast, colon, uterine, leukemia)	Neutral[9,17] or increased[9–11,17] Villareal—breast only
Cardiovascular morbidity (myocardial infarction, stroke)	Increased[9,17]
Cognitive function	Inconsistent[4,18]
Depression	Neutral[4,9]
Disability	Increased[4,19]
Osteoporosis and related fracture	Decreased[9,17,19]
Medication burden (no. of medications)	Increased[4,17]
Metabolic syndrome/ diabetes mellitus	Increased[9–11,17,19]
Mobility	Decreased[17]
Osteoarthritis	Increased[10,11,19]
Quality of life	Decreased[4]

Data from Refs.[4,9–11,17–19]

increased BMI reduces fracture risk at the hip and wrist. An increased BMI, however, increases risk of fracture in obese women at the ankle, lower leg, humerus, and spine.[23] Severe obesity associated with reduced mobility has a negative impact on bone density.[21]

OBESITY-RELATED RISKS THAT MATTER: IMPAIRED PHYSICAL FUNCTION AND FRAILTY

Obesity in late life confers a higher risk for impaired physical function,[1,7,10,11,15,24,25] a critically relevant outcome for older adults. Functional limitation is a mediator for poor quality of life.[1,7,10,11] Obese disabled patients frequently have muscle weakness, poor mobility, and higher fall rates.[5,10,11,24] Chronic pain[7,24] and other comorbidities (arthritis, cognitive impairment) seen with aging impart further physical limitations, which amplify the functional losses. Obesity potentiates frailty,[10,11,15,25] a decrease in strength, endurance, and physiologic function, and results in decreased physical reserves and increased vulnerability to injury and disability.[26] Although frailty is usually accompanied by weight loss and malnutrition, a study of acutely hospitalized patients older than 75 years of age identified 60% of normal weight, 42% of overweight, and 40% of obese patients as malnourished by Mini Nutritional Assessment score.[16]

WEIGHT LOSS FOR OLDER ADULTS: KEY MANAGEMENT POINTS

- Lifestyle modifications for weight loss are achievable and safe in older adults.
- Modest intentional weight loss is associated with significant improvements in quality of life and physical function.
- Moderate physical activity should be incorporated into all weight loss programs to maintain muscle mass, strength, bone density, balance, and functional status.

There have been few rigorous trials of weight loss treatments, particularly pharmacologic and surgical approaches, in elderly patients.[6,8,27] These studies are mostly short term (less than 1 year of follow-up) and focus primarily on lifestyle interventions.[6] Weight loss is accompanied by decreases in fat free mass in elderly patients.[6] Approximately 25% of weight lost is lean body mass, both bone mineral density and muscle mass.[15] Patients exhibiting rollercoaster weight changes (loss followed by regain, followed by loss) have more losses in lean muscle mass than if weight had remained stable[8]; this deters some providers from routinely recommending a weight loss regimen to obese older patients. In addition, there is no agreed on optimal BMI for the elderly. Recommending weight loss for elderly patients, therefore, must be individualized, recognizing and respecting each patient's goals of care, quality of life, and physical function.[9]

LIFESTYLE INTERVENTIONS FOR ELDERLY PATIENTS

Despite the known effect on lean body mass, weight loss therapy improves physical function and muscle quality.[6] Systematic reviews show late-life lifestyle interventions result in weight loss of up to 10% at 3 to 12 months.[6] A meta-analysis of weight loss interventions in adults over the age of 60 found that although a 3-kg weight loss at 1 year was achievable, there were no consistent patient-oriented outcomes.[27] As little as a 2-kg loss, or 3% of total body weight over 6 months, improves some cardiovascular and diabetes endpoints.[9] Improvements in physical function are seen with a weight loss of 3 to 4 kg over one to 3 years.[17] A 10% weight loss over 3 to 12 months improves physical function, metabolic outcomes, and cardiovascular risks in frail obese older adults.[6] A weight loss of 1 to 2 lb/wk or 8% to 10% over 6 months is achievable by reducing energy intake by 500 to 1000 kcal/d.[10,11] Nutrient deficiencies are more common in dieting elderly patients and must be accounted for in any reduced-calorie regimens.[8] In particular, consider calcium and vitamin D supplementation to ameliorate any negative impact on bone mineral density seen with voluntary weight loss.[6] Higher-protein diets are helpful for satiating qualities and to minimize muscle mass loss.[15,28,29]

Physical activity and resistance training are important to include in any comprehensive weight management program for older obese patients, particularly those with decreased lean body mass (sarcopenic obesity). Including aerobic training, resistance training, and balance activities improves function[6,8,10,11,25] and can result in significant quality-of-life gains and improved functional independence whether weight loss is achieved or not.

PHARMACOLOGIC MANAGEMENT

No medications for the treatment of obesity have been studied specifically in older adults, although trials of orlistat (Xenical)[8] and Qsymia[30] (a phentermine and topiramate combination) did not exclude participants based on age. Liraglutide (Victoza), a potent glucagon-like peptide receptor agonist that causes weight loss in diabetic patients, is a second- or third-line antidiabetic agent and has been studied in participants as old as 80 years.[7] There are not enough data to assess whether geriatric patients respond differently to any of these agents compared with other trial subjects. Many elderly patients are on a variety of medications. The addition of an obesity medication may compound polypharmacy issues and increase the risk of drug interactions. Weight loss medications can have significant side effects and should be used with caution in older adults.

SURGICAL MANAGEMENT

Bariatric surgery is traditionally reserved for patients under the age of 60 due to concerns of surgical risk and secondary complications. With improved mortality rates in the United States and United Kingdom, however, this trend may be changing.[7] Very few controlled trials have examined bariatric surgical outcomes in patients greater than the age of 65. Based on this limited data, older adults do have a higher rate of surgical complications and greater length of hospital stay.[8] Bariatric surgery, which usually causes rapid, extensive weight loss, may come at the expense of considerable disruption in everyday life for older individuals. Patient selection should consider preoperative functional independence and adaptability to changes in eating and bowel habits as well as the impact of potential immobilization on overall health during surgical recovery.[7] Quality of life and physical function outcomes following bariatric surgery in the elderly are limited. There is no current consensus about safety, age cutoff, and preferred bariatric procedure for older adults.

SUMMARY

Obesity is associated with functional limitations, which impact the older adult's quality of life. Much of the morbidity and mortality of excess adiposity in the elderly is unclear, partly because of inadequate measurement methods. Select patients may benefit from a weight loss plan incorporating a protein-enriched diet and an exercise regimen emphasizing resistance training. Pharmacologic and surgical management of geriatric obesity is generally not advisable due to the lack of available evidence and concerns for adverse effects. Obese elderly are a rising demographic and an important focus for further research.

REFERENCES

1. Mathus-Vliegen EM. Obesity and the elderly. J Clin Gastroenterol 2012;46(7): 533–44.
2. National Institutes of Health, National Heart, Lung, and Blood Institute. Managing overweight and obesity in adults: systematic evidence review from the obesity expert panel. 2013. Available at: http://www.nhlbi.nih.gov/health-pro/guidelines/in-develop/obesity-evidence-review. Accessed June 14, 2015.
3. World Health Organization. Global health risks: mortality and burden of disease attributable to selected major risks. 2009. Available at: http://www.who.int/healthinfo/global_burden_disease/GlobalHealthRisks_report_full.pdf. Accessed June 12, 2015.
4. Oreopoulos A, Kalantar-Zadeh K, Sharma AM, et al. The obesity paradox in the elderly: potential mechanisms and clinical implications. Clin Geriatr Med 2009; 25(4):643–59.
5. Waters DL, Baumgartner RN. Sarcopenia and obesity. Clin Geriatr Med 2011; 27(3):401–21.
6. Waters DL, Ward AL, Villareal DT. Weight loss in obese adults 65 years and older: a review of the controversy. Exp Gerontol 2013;48(10):1054–61.
7. Han TS, Wu FC, Lean ME. Obesity and weight management in the elderly: a focus on men. Best Pract Res Clin Endocrinol Metab 2013;27(4):509–25.
8. Felix HC, West DS. Effectiveness of weight loss interventions for obese older adults. Am J Health Promot 2013;27(3):191–9.
9. Bales CW, Buhr G. Is obesity bad for older persons? A systematic review of the pros and cons of weight reduction in later life. J Am Med Dir Assoc 2008;9(5):302–12.
10. Villareal DT, Apovian CM, Kushner RF, et al. Obesity in older adults: technical review and position statement of the American Society for Nutrition and NAASO, the Obesity Society. Am J Clin Nutr 2005;82:923–34.
11. National Institutes of Health, National Heart, Lung, and Blood Institute. Executive summary of the clinical guidelines on the identification, evaluation, and treatment of overweight and obesity in adults. Arch Intern Med 1998;158:1855–67.
12. Alam I, Ng TP, Larbi A. Does inflammation determine whether obesity is metabolically healthy or unhealthy? The aging perspective. Mediators Inflamm 2012; 2012:456456.
13. Heiat A, Vaccarino V, Krumholz HM. An evidence-based assessment of federal guidelines for overweight and obesity as they apply to elderly persons. Arch Intern Med 2001;161(9):1194–203.
14. Donini LM, Savina C, Gennaro E, et al. A systematic review of the literature concerning the relationship between obesity and mortality in the elderly. J Nutr Health Aging 2012;16(1):89–98.
15. Mathus-Vliegen L, Toouli J, Fried M, et al. World Gastroenterology Organisation global guidelines on obesity. J Clin Gastroenterol 2012;46(7):555–61.
16. Lang PO, Mahmoudi R, Novella JL, et al. Is obesity a marker of robustness in vulnerable hospitalized aged populations? Prospective, multicenter cohort study of 1 306 acutely ill patients. J Nutr Health Aging 2014;18(1):66–74.
17. McTigue KM, Hess R, Ziouras J. Obesity in older adults: a systematic review of the evidence for diagnosis and treatment. Obesity 2006;14:1485–97.

18. Luchsinger JA, Cheng D, Tang MX, et al. Central obesity in the elderly is related to late-onset Alzheimer disease. Alzheimer Dis Assoc Disord 2012;26(2):101–5.

19. Janssen I. Morbidity and mortality risk associated with an overweight BMI in older men and women. Obesity (Silver Spring) 2007;15:1827–40.

20. Thomas F, Pannier B, Benetos A, et al. Visceral obesity is not an independent risk factor of mortality in subjects over 65 years. Vasc Health Risk Manag 2013;9: 739–45.

21. Zanandrea V, Barreto de Souto P, Cesari M, et al. Obesity and nursing home: a review and update. Clin Nutr 2013;32(5):679–85.

22. Visvanathan R, Haywood C, Piantadosi C, et al. Australian and New Zealand Society for Geriatric Medicine: position statement—obesity and the older person. Australas J Ageing 2012;31(4):261–7.

23. Compston JE, Flahive J, Hooven FH, et al. Obesity, health-care utilization, and health-related quality of life after fracture in postmenopausal women: Global Longitudinal Study of Osteoporosis in Women (GLOW). Calcif Tissue Int 2014;94(2): 223–31.

24. Fowler-Brown A, Wee CC, Marcantonio E, et al. The mediating effect of chronic pain on the relationship between obesity and physical function and disability in older adults. J Am Geriatr Soc 2013;61(12):2079–86.

25. Porter Starr KN, McDonald SR, Bales CW. Obesity and physical frailty in older adults: a scoping review of lifestyle intervention trials. J Am Med Dir Assoc 2014;15(4):240–50.

26. Morley JE, Vellas B, van Kan A, et al. Frailty consensus: a call to action. J Am Med Dir Assoc 2013;14:392–7.

27. Witham MD, Avenell A. Interventions to achieve long-term weight loss in obese older people: a systematic review and meta-analysis. Age Ageing 2010;39(2): 176–84.

28. Du Y, Ou H, Beverly EA, et al. Achieving glycemic control in elderly patients with type 2 diabetes: a critical comparison of current options. Clin Interv Aging 2014; 9:1963–80.

29. Li Z, Heber D. Sarcopenic obesity in the elderly and strategies for weight management. Nutr Rev 2012;70(1):57–64.

30. Food and Drug Administration. Highlights of prescribing information: Qysmia. 2014. Available at: http://www.accessdata.fda.gov/drugsatfda_docs/label/2014/022580s010s011s012lbl.pdf. Accessed on June 13, 2015.

Surgical Management of Metabolic Syndrome Related to Morbid Obesity

Scott T. Rehrig Jr, MD

KEYWORDS

- Morbid obesity • Metabolic surgery • Multimodal surgical pathway
- Surgical outcomes • Surgical risk • Bile acids • Gut microbiome

KEY POINTS

- Morbid obesity and metabolic syndrome are a global epidemic.
- The limited efficacy of intensive medical therapy is related to complex socioeconomic and biologic factors that cause most individuals to regain weight.
- Prerequisites for metabolic surgery include medical, nutrition, and behavioral assessments to ensure patients are medically optimized and mentally and emotionally prepared for the postoperative period.
- The understanding of the mechanisms of action of metabolic surgery has evolved from restriction and malabsorption to the complex interaction of neurologic and enteric hormones, changes in gut biochemical pathways, and the important role of the gut microbiome.

INTRODUCTION

The World Health Organization has invoked the term "globesity" to describe the worldwide epidemic of obesity. In 2014, nearly 2 billion individuals worldwide were overweight (body mass index [BMI], 25–30 kg/m^2). A total of 600 million individuals were obese (BMI >30 kg/m^2). The worldwise rise of obesity creates a paradox of malnutrition and obesity occurring side by side in the same country. With rising global sourcing of inexpensive processed foods (of poor nutritional value) it is difficult for many individuals to consume an affordable, balanced, and nutritious diet. Overconsumption of processed foods contributes to obesity and the metabolic syndrome.[1,2] Metabolic syndrome is defined as a combination of diabetes plus two of any of the following: morbid obesity (BMI >30 kg/m^2), hypertension, hypertriglyceridemia, or hypercholesterolemia.

Morbid obesity is historically resistant to treatment and may not be curable. The annual probability of a morbidly obese (BMI ≥40 kg/m^2) person obtaining a normal

Uniformed Services University of the Health Sciences, Bethesda, MD, USA
E-mail address: scott.rehrig@usuhs.edu

Prim Care Clin Office Pract 43 (2016) 145–158
http://dx.doi.org/10.1016/j.pop.2015.10.003   **primarycare.theclinics.com**
0095-4543/16/$ – see front matter Published by Elsevier Inc.

weight with medical therapy is 1 in 1290 for males and 1 in 677 for females.[3] The annual probability of achieving 5% weight reduction is one in eight for males and one in seven for females.[3] Most weight loss programs, therefore, currently recommend a 5% to 10% reduction in weight as a target goal.

Beyond the obvious health consequences, morbid obesity also has an enormous economic impact. In the United States, morbid obesity increases direct medical costs by 42%.[4] Annual health care expenditures to treat morbid obesity–related diseases approach nearly $150 billion per year.[4] Obesity also impacts national security. In one study, 27% of draft-eligible US adults age 17 to 24 were deemed unfit for military service because of weight-related restrictions.[5] In the US military health care system (one of largest health care systems in world, providing care to more than 9 million patients) roughly 70% of the beneficiaries are overweight or obese.[5]

Current treatment approaches in morbid obesity are multimodal in nature. Combination therapies include increases in moderate-intensity aerobic and resistance exercise; behavioral lifestyle changes to increase compliance with diet and activity recommendations; medical nutrition therapy (including diets with energy deficits >500 kcal per day); intensive medical therapy (pharmacologic treatment of cardiovascular comorbidities and possible prescription of weight loss medications); and (increasingly) metabolic surgical procedures, such as gastric bypass and vertical sleeve gastrectomy (VSG). Each of these therapies attempts to mitigate the metabolic consequences of obesity.[6] This article focuses on the preoperative evaluation and proper patient selection for metabolic surgery. The procedures are discussed relative to their anatomy, metabolic mechanism of action, and common adverse effects.

PRESURGERY MEDICAL EVALUATION

The preoperative evaluation and selection of metabolic surgery patients is best done by a multidisciplinary team. Standard components of the preoperative examination include a full medical assessment with risk stratification, nutritional counseling, and behavioral health evaluation and support. Most health care systems use a checklist or algorithmic approach to preoperative management based on a centers of excellence model with existing best practices.

The medical evaluation includes a complete history and physical focusing on obesity-related comorbidities, documenting weight, height, and BMI. The history should include prior attempts at self or medically directed weight loss. Laboratory evaluations should include a complete chemical profile including liver and kidney functions, fasting blood glucose, hemoglobin A_{1c}, and a lipid profile. Blood type, coagulation profile, and hemoglobin (Hb) levels are assessed. Micronutrient measurements include iron stores, vitamin B_{12}, folate, and vitamin D levels. Deficiencies should be corrected preoperatively.

Patients with a BMI greater than 35 kg/m^2 have a high incidence of obstructive sleep apnea (OSA). OSA is associated with major cardiopulmonary morbidity. Controversy exists as to the whether or not all bariatric patients should undergo polysomnography testing. OSA screening and confirmatory polysomnography should be performed preoperatively. The use of continuous positive airway pressure in the perioperative period may decrease cardiopulmonary morbidity. The American Society for Metabolic and Bariatric Surgery (ASMBS) and the Society for Gastrointestinal and Endoscopic Surgeons recommend that all patients diagnosed with moderate to severe OSA use continuous positive airway pressure preoperatively and in the immediate postoperative period.[7,8]

PRESURGERY NUTRITIONAL ASSESSMENT AND EDUCATION

Metabolic surgery patients must undergo thorough presurgery nutritional education and training to prepare them for postoperative dietary success. Nutritional deficiencies and malnutrition are major risk factors long term after metabolic surgery. Nutritional education, therefore, is essential for postsurgical success. There is little consensus, however, as to the best mode or duration of perioperative nutritional education. Individualized, group, or World Wide Web–based learning modalities are all available. Many presurgical nutritional algorithms are driven by insurance plans and institutional preference. Some bariatric programs require patients to adhere to individual and group therapy sessions organized by medical nutritionists for at least 3 months before surgery. Other programs ask patients to participate in 6 months of a physician-supervised medical weight loss program.

Weight loss surgery patients must also be informed about changes in their ability to eat postoperatively. Nutrition support programs review necessary postoperative changes to macronutrient and micronutrient intake, postoperative eating strategies, and the need for frequent fluid intake. Medical nutritionists should be directly involved in the preoperative patient assessment and render an opinion about each patient's candidacy for surgery. If the nutritionist does not believe a patient is adequately prepared to make the necessary behavior changes to successfully live with dietary changes mandated by their bariatric surgery, then the procedure should be delayed or even avoided. Some programs use objective tests to assess the patient's preparation for surgery from a nutritional perspective.

One of the key goals of the presurgical nutritional assessment is to identify preexisting micronutrient deficiencies (because metabolic surgeries often exacerbate such deficits postoperatively). Vitamin D, magnesium, phosphate, iron, and vitamin A deficiencies are the most common.[9] Higher preoperative BMI correlates with an increased risk for deficiency.[9] One common practice is to start patients on daily multivitamin supplement along with calcium citrate and vitamin D (1200 mg/400 IU).

Another common requirement in many metabolic surgery programs is preoperative weight loss. Although widespread in implementation, the practice is debatable. ASMBS guidelines weakly recommend the practice, whereas others suggest that focusing on preoperative weight loss may actually harm patients already at high risk for malnutrition because of dysfunctional eating behaviors.[10] When preoperative weight loss is desired, patients are generally placed on a high-protein, low-carbohydrate diet (1000–1200 kcals/day) using commercial meal replacement products 2 weeks before surgery. The intent is to improve intraoperative management of an enlarged liver often encountered during laparoscopy in the morbidly obese patient. A liquid diet shrinks the volume of the liver by depleting fat and glycogen stores thereby improving visualization at the esophagogastric junction.[10,11]

During the early and long-term postoperative period, frequent medical nutrition follow-up is essential to reinforce newly learned eating behaviors and to help patients through a period of "surgically induced starvation." Guidelines recommend a minimum of every 3 month nutrition follow-up with frequent macronutrient and micronutrient assessments[10,11] (Table 1). Regardless of the degree of preoperative preparation, patients require frequent and ongoing nutritional and psychological support. Group support meetings are an efficient way to provide postoperative care. Patients who attend greater numbers of postoperative visits seem to have superior long-term weight loss.[11]

Table 1
Preoperative and postoperative evaluation after laparoscopic Roux-en-Y gastric bypass, laparoscopic sleeve gastrectomy, and biliopancreatic diversion with duodenal switch: 2013 recommendations of the SMOB

	Preop	2 wk	4 wk	6 wk	8 wk	3 mo	6 mo	9 mo	1 y	1½ y	2 y	2½ y	3 y	3½ y	4 y	4½ y	5 y
Radiology																	
DEXA											a		a		a		a
Laboratory Testing																	
Hemogram																	
INR/Quick																	
Sedimentation Rate																	
C-reactive Protein																	
Potassium																	
Calcium																	
Urinary calcium						a		a			a		a		a		a
Magnesium								a			a		a	a	a		a
Phosphorus																	
Iron									a		a		a		a		a
Zinc									a		a		a		a		a
Glucose																	
Creatinin																	
Transferrin																	
Ferritin																	
Transthyretin						a	a		a		a		a		a		a
Vitamin A/cis-Retinol						b	b		b		b		b		b		b
Vitamin E																	
Vitamin D3/25-OH-calciferol																	
Vitamin B1																	
Vitamin B2																	
Vitamin B6																	
Vitamin B12																	
Holotranscobalamine																	
Folic acid in erythrocytes																	
Parathormone																	

SMOB-recommendations :

Mandatory	■
Helpful	▨
Not recommended	☐

SMOB (www.smob.ch) recommendations were established from the recommendations stated by the American Association of Clinical Endocrinologists, the American Society for Metabolic and Bariatric Surgery, and The Obesity Society. SMOB gave recommendations until the fifth postoperative year. However, many experts recommend a life-long monitoring.

Abbreviations: DEXA, dual X-ray energy absorptiometry; SMOB, Swiss Society for the Study of Morbid Obesity and Metabolic Disorders.

[a] For laparoscopic Roux-en-Y gastric bypass and biliopancreatic diversion with duodenal switch patients.

[b] For biliopancreatic diversion with duodenal switch patients only.

From Thibault R, Huber O, Azagury DE, et al. Twelve key nutritional issues in bariatric surgery. Clin Nutr 2015 Mar 3. http://dx.doi.org/10.1016/j.clnu.2015.02.012. [Epub ahead of print].

PRESURGERY PSYCHOLOGICAL ASSESSMENT

Current National Institutes of Health, ASMBS, and International Federation for the Surgery of Obesity and Metabolic Disorders guidelines strongly recommended that candidates for metabolic surgery undergo a behavioral health evaluation before surgery.[11–13] The goal of this evaluation is to diagnose and treat underlying behavioral disorders that may negatively impact short- and long-term outcomes. Twenty percent of metabolic surgery patients have underlying behavioral health diagnoses including affective disorders (anxiety, depression), personality disorders, eating behavior disorders, and low self-esteem.[14]

Guidelines also recommend that the preoperative evaluation include an assessment of patient expectations from the surgery, an eating behavior history, an assessment of self-motivation, a screening for substance abuse, and an overview of the patient's familial support structure. Despite these recommendations, results are mixed as to the impact of preoperative treatment of behavioral health disorders on long-term success with weight management.[15] One meta-analysis notes positive effects of behavioral intervention and support group attendance on patient outcomes.[15] A second meta-analysis found that a history of binge eating negatively affects metabolic surgery outcomes. Surprisingly, such variables as depression, anxiety, prior sexual abuse, and alcohol abuse were not convincingly correlated with metabolic surgery outcomes.[16] Both reports note significant heterogeneity of data, poor follow-up, and cite the need for more rigorous future research.[15,16]

WHY MEDICALLY SUPERVISED TREATMENT FAILS

To date, medically directed weight loss programs have met with limited success as a means to treat metabolic syndrome. It seems that once the body gains significant fat stores, it tenaciously defends these stores.[17] When placed on a calorie-restricted diet as part of medical weight loss therapy, a complex system of hormones signal the body to feed to replace the lost energy stores. This may explain why so many individuals regain weight after initial success with dieting. This response also makes sense from an evolutionary standpoint in the context of survival and reproduction.[17]

Other biologic factors, such as adipose cellularity, endocrine function, energy metabolism, and neural responsivity, contribute to weight gain after dieting. Obese individuals have increased fat mass and increased numbers of adipose cells. Medical treatment shrinks the fat mass but not the number of fat cells. After medically induced weight loss, it is normal for adipose cells to signal the body to replenish their fat stores. This process (likely mediated by leptin) functions to prevent starvation. In the medical weight loss patient, leptin levels are suppressed. This results in lower energy expenditure, increased hunger, reduced thyroid metabolism, and diminished sympathetic nervous activity.[18] These factors combine to promote weight regain rather than help to maintain loss.

Other neurobiologic mechanisms further complicate patient efforts to sustain weight loss. Food intake is neurologic, regulated by three interconnected systems: (1) homeostatic, (2) reward, and (3) inhibition. The reward system, a dopaminergic mesolimbic pathway, is upregulated by diets high in processed sugar, salt, and fats. Over time, dopaminergic pathways are downregulated by habituation. This means that individuals require increasingly larger stimuli (eg, processed foods) to reap the same reward. This is analogous to neural processes noted in other addictive behaviors. During intensive behavioral weight loss therapy, patients are able to overcome this habituated state. When behavioral therapy ceases, however, many individuals struggle to restrain previously upregulated reward pathways and revert to behaviors that result in weight gain.[18]

Given the vast lay literature recommending certain macronutrient diets, another interesting study suggests that the mix of macronutrients in a diet is less important than calorie restriction. Over 800 individuals were assigned to one of four diets varying in protein, fat, and carbohydrate ratios. Subjects were followed for 2 years. All participants were calorie restricted by a net deficit of 750 calories per day from their normal baseline. In this trial, macronutrient composition did not determine outcome. All four diets equally demonstrated an average of 4 kg of weight loss after 2 years of follow-up. Importantly, support group attendance correlated strongly with weight loss for each diet type.[19]

MECHANISMS OF ACTION OF METABOLIC SURGERY

Metabolic surgery exerts its effects through weight-dependent and weight-independent mechanisms. The BRAVE mechanism (Bile flow alteration, Reduction gastric volume, Anatomic rearrangement/Altered flow nutrients, Vagal manipulation, Enteric gut hormones) has been used to describe the effects of metabolic surgery.[20] In addition to the drastic reduction in gastric volumes created by metabolic surgery (weight-dependent effects), two areas of weight-independent effects under intense study are alterations in bile acid physiology and changes in the gut microbiome.

The physiologic changes in bile acids seen after gastric bypass have been described by the mnemonic SLIMMER (Satiety, Lipid and cholesterol metabolism, Incretins and glucose homeostasis, energy Metabolism, gut Microbiome, Endoplasmic Reticulum stress). After gastric bypass, bile acid flow is increased to the terminal ileum where TGR5 receptor activation leads to the increased secretion of glucagon-like peptide 1 (GLP-1).[20] GLP-1, an incretin, promotes insulin secretion and inhibits glucagon function yielding a net decrease in blood glucose concentration. The increased secretion of GLP-1 is an example of the how gastric bypass exhibits a positive incretin effect via changes in bile acid flow.[20]

Animal models further clarify the understanding of bile acid physiology and the metabolic syndrome. One study assessed the effects of diverting bile acid flow to different parts of the small intestine in a rodent model. In diet-induced diabetic rodents, anastomosis of the gallbladder to the ileum resulted in sustained weight loss, improved glucose tolerance, and decreased triglyceride parameters similar to gastric bypass.[21]

Research into the gut microbiome in morbidly obese patients is also yielding insights into how the gut flora influences the pathophysiology of the metabolic syndrome. The host colonic gut microbiome affects metabolic disease through digestion of carbohydrates into short chain fatty acids, such as acetate, propionate, and butyrate. These short-chain fatty acids lead to the secretion of incretins, such as peptide YY and GLP-1, which further promotes reductions in host energy uptake and improves insulin sensitivity.[22]

Studies of the gut microbiome in gastric bypass patients demonstrate decreases in the ratio of Firmicutes/Bacteroidetes and increases in Proteobacteria species. As a comparison, medical weight loss studies note similar changes in Firmicutes/Bacteroidetes ratios but not the increases in Proteobacteria. A randomized trial of gastric bypass patients demonstrated improved surgical weight loss outcomes in the group given oral *Lactobacillus* probiotic supplements compared with a standard postoperative protocol. It was hypothesized that bile acids have direct incretin effects (improving glucose sensitivity) and indirect effects mediated by gut microbiome (eg, Proteobacteria) via a feedforward mechanism.[23]

Bile acid and microbiome studies are only beginning to unravel complex effects that metabolic surgeries have on the gut-liver axis. Although these studies improve the current understanding of the pathophysiology of the metabolic syndrome and obesity, they also highlight the multimodal nature of metabolic syndrome and the need for future research.

METABOLIC SURGERY OUTCOMES

Historically there have been few high-quality randomized controlled trials examining the practice of metabolic surgery. Two recent trials highlight the effectiveness of metabolic surgery. The STAMPEDE trial compared Roux-en-Y gastric bypass (RYGB) and VSG with intensive medical therapy for morbid obesity patients with uncontrolled type

2 diabetes. At 3 years of follow-up, the primary end point (HbA_{1c} of 6% or less) was reached by 5% of the medical therapy group and 38% of RYGB group ($P = .01$).[24] A similar trial randomized patients to surgery versus intensive medical therapy for type 2 diabetes. A primary outcome was the partial ($HbA_{1c} <6.5\%$) or complete ($HbA_{1c} <5.7\%$) remission of diabetes. In this trial, 40% patients who underwent RYGB had partial remission, whereas 15% demonstrated complete resolution of diabetes after 3 years of follow-up. No patients in the medical treatment group demonstrated partial or complete remission.[25]

The Swedish Obesity Study, a prospective case-control trial, represents the most comprehensive evaluation of the effects metabolic surgery to date. The primary end point of the study was mortality. Surgical patients experienced a 30% reduction in mortality compared with medical treatment at Year 13 of the study. Secondary end points were diabetes remission and prevention. At 2 and 10 years, surgical patients demonstrated diabetes remission rates of 72% and 35%, respectively. Metabolic surgery reduced the incidence of diabetes by 84% and 78% at 10 and 15 years, respectively.[26]

A systematic review of nearly 8000 patients who underwent metabolic surgery from 1946 through 2014 noted diabetes remission of rates ($HbA_{1c} <6.5\%$) of up to 66%, remission rates of 38% for hypertension, and remission rates of up to 60% for hyperlipidemia following gastric bypass.[27] Another systematic review reported remission rates of 92% (95% confidence interval, 85%–97%) for diabetes, 75% (95% confidence interval, 62%–86%) for hypertension, and 76% (95% confidence interval, 56%–91%) for dyslipidemia in patients undergoing gastric bypass.[28]

SURGICAL TREATMENT OPTIONS

Bariatric surgery is an effective (and some would argue, underused) treatment of metabolic syndrome. In 2013, for example, approximately 0.01% of the total estimated population of morbid obese surgical candidates underwent a metabolic procedure.[29] The most common procedure worldwide was the RYGB (45%). This was followed by the VSG (37%). A laparoscopic approach was used for most (96%) metabolic surgical procedures. Robotic-assisted techniques are available, but represent the minority of the cases performed internationally.[29]

Roux-en-Y Gastric Bypass

Overall the RYGB remains the gold standard for metabolic surgery. It is the most commonly performed procedure and has the longest outcomes data.[29] The operation is performed laparoscopically through six small incisions ranging in size from 5 to 12 mm.

During the construction of the RYGB, a small (30 mL) gastric pouch is connected to an antecolic, antegastric limb of jejunum (the Roux limb), which is 125 to 150 cm long. The remnant stomach, biliary system, and pancreas drain through the biliopancreatic limb and converge with the Roux limb at an anastomosis approximately 50 cm distal to the ligament of Treitz. The small intestine beyond the anastomosis is called the common channel. It is this region of the small intestine where the mixing of bypassed nutrients, and pancreatic and biliary secretions occurs (**Fig. 1**).

Vertical Sleeve Gastrectomy

The VSG is the second most commonly performed bariatric operation in the world. More than 170,000 procedures were performed in 2013.[29] The operation is performed laparoscopically through five or six small incisions ranging in size from 5 to 12 mm. During

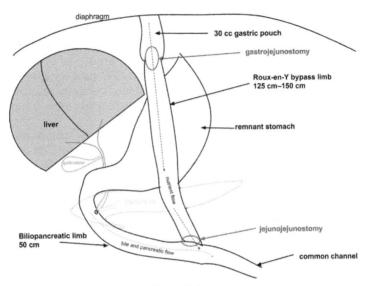

Fig. 1. Antecolic, antegastric, Roux-en-Y gastric bypass.

the formation of a VSG, 80% of the stomach (fundus, body, and some antrum) is resected with a bariatric endoscopic stapler using a bougie as a guide to limit luminal stenosis and maintain symmetry. The vascular supply to the sleeve originates from the vessels of the lesser gastric curvature. The VSG is approximately 1 to 2 cm in diameter and 8 cm in length. The pylorus is spared with variable amounts of the antrum. Nutrients flow aborally through the restrictive sleeve and out the pylorus (**Fig. 2**).

The mechanisms of action of the VSG in terms of weight loss are (1) the mechanical restriction of the sleeve, (2) putative physiologic effects related to the resection of the

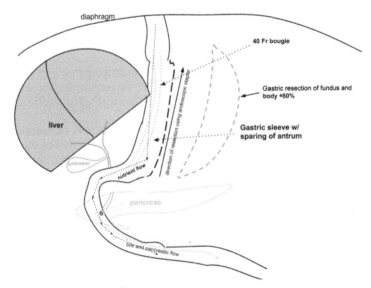

Fig. 2. A 40F catheter vertical sleeve gastrectomy.

gastric fundus containing ghrelin cells, and (3) possibly increased motility of nutrients into the small intestine. Decreased levels of ghrelin, an appetite-promoting hormone and activator of the dopaminergic mesolimbic reward system of the brain, have been consistently noted post-VSG. Decreased ghrelin levels may also contribute to the anorexia VSG patients experience postoperatively. An incretin effect has also been noted after VSG. Increased levels of GLP-1 have been reported and may contribute to the improvement of diabetes post-VSG.[30–32]

Adjustable Gastric Banding

Adjustable gastric banding (AGB) accounts for 10% of all bariatric procedures, making it the third most commonly performed bariatric operation in the world. More than 45,000 AGB procedures were reported in 2013.[29] The AGB consists of a silicon backbone, a soft balloon that sits in circumferential contact with the stomach, and a tube connecting the balloon to an access port, which is placed on the anterior abdominal wall. The surgeon places the band around the stomach approximately 1 to 2 cm distal to the gastroesophageal junction and secures the band in place by performing an anterior gastrogastric plication[32] (**Fig. 3**). The mechanism of action of the AGB is purely restrictive, based on the volume of fluid injected into the balloon reservoir.

Biliopancreatic Diversion with Duodenal Switch

Biliopancreatic diversion with duodenal switch (BPD/DS) is a highly specialized metabolic surgery performed in international centers of excellence. This procedure represents approximately 3% of all worldwide metabolic surgeries.[29] The BPD/DS is the

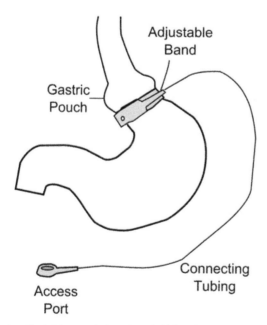

Fig. 3. Laparoscopic adjustable gastric band. A rigid band with an inflatable balloon lining the inner aspect is placed around the upper stomach. The band is tightened by injecting saline into the subcutaneous access port. Most surgeons in the United States secure the band anteriorly by using two to five sutures to imbricate the stomach over the band, not shown in this diagram. (*Courtesy of* Daniel M. Herron, MD, New York, NY.)

most efficacious metabolic surgery, consistently leading to more than 80% excess weight loss and near complete resolution of the metabolic syndrome. It is not widely performed in the United States because of the technical demands and the sophisti-cated level of care that is required to support patients in the perioperative period. The BPD/DS consists of a VSG that is anastomosed to a 250- to 300-cm alimentary limb diverting nutrients away from the proximal small intestine. Undigested nutrients mix with bile and pancreatic secretions in a 100-cm common channel creating true malabsorption of macronutrients and micronutrients[32] (**Fig. 4**). The BDP/DS exerts similar effects on the enteric gut hormones as the RYGB.

SURGICAL COMPLICATIONS

Metabolic surgery is safe and highly effective. A review of 29 prospective studies with 8000 metabolic surgery patients noted a mortality rate of 1% for gastric bypass.[27] A second review of nearly 4000 patients from 10 US health care systems showed a 90-day postoperative mortality rate of 0.4%. The Obesity Surgery Mortality Risk Score (OS-MRS) risk factors of BMI greater than or equal to 50 kg/m^2, male sex, age greater than or equal to 45 years, hypertension, and risk of pulmonary embolism (prior diag-nosis chronic venous stasis, inferior vena cava filter, pulmonary embolism, or obesity hypoventilation syndrome) were validated in this study. The OS-MRS is a helpful tool

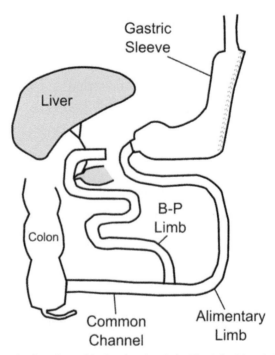

Fig. 4. Biliopancreatic diversion with duodenal switch. The left side of the stomach is re-sected, forming a sleeve gastrectomy. The duodenum is divided just distal to the pylorus and connected to the ileum. The remainder of the duodenum and jejunum pass only bile and pancreatic juice; this bypassed intestine is referred to as the biliopancreatic (B-P) limb. The only area where ingested food and digestive juices intermix is the common chan-nel, generally the distalmost 50 to 125 cm of ileum. (*Courtesy of* Daniel M. Herron, MD, New York, NY.)

to distinguish high-risk surgical candidates. Using OS-MRS criteria, only 4% of the study population was deemed high-risk. These individuals had a 21-fold risk of death compared with the low-risk group.[33]

The common metabolic surgical procedures seem to be safe. Courcoulas and colleagues[25] reported minimal morbidity and no mortality in either surgical arm of their randomized controlled trial at 3 years. Schauer and colleagues[24] reported complications from the STAMPEDE study (randomized controlled trial, RYGB vs VSG vs medical therapy, N = 150), but noted no deaths and no life-threatening adverse events at 3 years.

POSTOPERATIVE CARE
Acute Phase (24–48 hours)

The care of the acute postsurgery metabolic patient involves multiple disciplines including nursing, medicine, physical therapy, and nutrition services. The surgical and nursing teams are mainly responsible for the acute postoperative period. Most routine cases of metabolic surgery require 1 or 2 days of hospitalization. Most institutions use protocols that emphasize early mobilization of patients to help minimize thromboembolic and pulmonary complications. Nausea is aggressively treated with scheduled antiemetic medication. Narcotics are minimized postoperatively because they impede return of gut function and are a major risk for respiratory complications.

Routine vital signs and pulse oximetry are monitored the first 24 hours. The physical examination of the postoperative metabolic surgery patient is unreliable. Sustained heart rate elevations greater than 110 to 120 beats per minute warrant urgent investigation, because this finding is a sensitive indicator of a possible adverse event. Metabolic surgeons often return patients to the operating room for laparoscopic exploration if there is a high suspicion for a gastrointestinal leak. Most institutions do not routinely obtain postoperative radiographic images unless a gastrointestinal leak or other acute event is suspected.

Patients are generally advanced to a full liquid diet within the first 24 hours following surgery. Patients are encouraged to frequently drink small sips (30–60 mL) to acclimate to postoperative changes in the volume of the gastric tract.

Medical management of diabetes and hypertension is often simplified because calorie restriction and the putative effects of the surgery have a rapid impact on glucose homeostasis. Most patients are able to resume oral medications at discharge.

Chronic Phase (1 month to 2 years)

Metabolic surgery mitigates but does not cure metabolic disease. Patients require lifelong multidisciplinary medical, nutritional, and psychosocial support to maintain and sustain the progress. Metabolic surgery is considered successful once patients obtain greater than or equal to 50% excess weight loss. Postsurgical failure to obtain greater than or equal to 50% excess weight loss or weight regain is expected in 20% to 30% of patients.[34] Patients who demonstrate the greatest long-term success ($\geq$50% excess weight loss) following surgery show moderate adherence to postsurgical eating behaviors, regular attendance at support group meetings, and limit grazing (snacking) behavior to no more than once per day.[34] Superobese patients (BMI >53 kg m²) demonstrated poorer outcomes.

SUMMARY/DISCUSSION

Worldwide, the prevalence of morbid obesity and metabolic syndrome continues to rise. The factors contributing to the lack of success of intensive behavioral-based therapies for metabolic syndrome are complex. They involve the interplay of socioeconomic and sophisticated evolutionarily based biologic systems that create the modern obesogenic environment.

Metabolic surgery represents the most efficacious means of treating the metabolic syndrome. Medical science and engineering have advanced the practice of metabolic surgery to the point where it has become routine and safe. The understanding of the mechanisms of action of metabolic surgery is evolving away from simple ideas of gastric restriction and nutrient malabsorption to a deeper understanding of the molecular interactions of neuro–gut hormone axes and the influence of the colonic microbiome. This increasing depth of understanding opens new avenues for investigation that are yielding new therapies and novel procedures such that in the future metabolic surgery, such as gastric bypass, may become obsolete. For the near future, surgeons will continue to advance the practice of metabolic surgery using evidence-based multimodal approaches and embracing new surgical technologies to minimize risk and maximize successful outcomes.

REFERENCES

1. World Health Organization. Controlling the global obesity epidemic. Available at: http://www.who.int/nutrition/topics/obesity/en/. Accessed August 6, 2015.
2. World Health Organization. Obesity and overweight. Available at: http://www.who.int/mediacentre/factsheets/fs311/en/. Accessed August 6, 2015.
3. Fildes A, Charlton J, Rudisill C, et al. Probability of an obese person attaining normal body weight: cohort study using electronic health records. Am J Public Health 2015;105(9):e54–9.
4. Finkelstein EA. How big of a problem is obesity? Surg Obes Relat Dis 2014;10(4): 569–70.
5. Tanofsky-Kraff M, Sbrocco T, Stephens MB, et al. Obesity and the US military family. Obesity (Silver Spring) 2013;21(11):2205–20.
6. Jensen MD, Ryan DH, Apovian CM, et al, American College of Cardiology/American Heart Association Task Force on Practice Guidelines; Obesity Society. 2013 AHA/ACC/TOS guideline for the management of overweight and obesity in adults: a report of the American College of Cardiology/American Heart Association Task Force on Practice Guidelines and The Obesity Society. J Am Coll Cardiol 2014;63(25 Pt B):2985–3023.
7. ASMBS Clinical Issues Committee. Perioperative management of obstructive sleep apnea. Surg Obes Relat Dis 2012;8(3):e27–32.
8. Shikora ST. Airway and sleep apnea perioperative consideration. SAGES website. Available at: http://www.sages.org/video/airway-and-sleep-apnea-perioperative-consideration. Accessed August 06, 2015.
9. Lefebvre P, Letois F, Sultan A, et al. Nutrient deficiencies in patients with obesity considering bariatric surgery: a cross-sectional study. Surg Obes Relat Dis 2014; 10(3):540–6.
10. Thibault R, Huber O, Azagury DE, et al. Twelve key nutritional issues in bariatric surgery. Clin Nutr 2015;34.
11. Mechanick JI, Youdim A, Jones DB, et al. Clinical practice guidelines for the perioperative nutritional, metabolic, and nonsurgical support of the bariatric surgery patient–2013 update: cosponsored by American Association of Clinical Endocrinologists, the Obesity Society, and American Society for Metabolic & Bariatric Surgery. Surg Obes Relat Dis 2013;9(2):159–91.

12. Fried M, Yumuk V, Oppert JM, et al, International Federation for Surgery of Obesity and Metabolic Disorders-European Chapter (IFSO-EC), European Association for the Study of Obesity (EASO), European Association for the Study of Obesity, Obesity Management Task Force (EASO OMTF). Interdisciplinary European guidelines on metabolic and bariatric surgery. Obes Surg 2014;24(1): 42–55.

13. Gastrointestinal Surgery for Severe Obesity. National Institutes of Health Consensus Development Conference Statement March 25-27, 1991. Available at: http://consensus.nih.gov/1991/1991GISurgeryObesity084html.htm. Accessed August 06, 2015.

14. Pull CB. Current psychological assessment practices in obesity surgery programs: what to assess and why. Curr Opin Psychiatry 2010;23(1):30–6.

15. Rudolph A, Hilbert A. Post-operative behavioural management in bariatric surgery: a systematic review and meta-analysis of randomized controlled trials. Obes Rev 2013;14(4):292–302.

16. Livhits M, Mercado C, Yermilov I, et al. Preoperative predictors of weight loss following bariatric surgery: systematic review. Obes Surg 2012;22(1):70–89.

17. Larder R, O'Rahilly S. Shedding pounds after going under the knife: guts over glory—why diets fail. Nat Med 2012;18(5):666–7.

18. Ochner CN, Barrios DM, Lee CD, et al. Biological mechanisms that promote weight regain following weight loss in obese humans. Physiol Behav 2013;120: 106–13.

19. Sacks FM, Bray GA, Carey VJ, et al. Comparison of weight-loss diets with different compositions of fat, protein, and carbohydrates. N Engl J Med 2009; 360(9):859–73.

20. Penney NC, Kinross J, Newton RC, et al. The role of bile acids in reducing the metabolic complications of obesity after bariatric surgery: a systematic review. Int J Obes (Lond) 2015;39(11):1565–74.

21. Flynn CR, Albaugh VL, Cai S, et al. Bile diversion to the distal small intestine has comparable metabolic benefits to bariatric surgery. Nat Commun 2015;6:7715.

22. Hur KY, Lee MS. Gut microbiome and metabolic disorders. Diabetes Metab J 2015;39(3):198–203.

23. Sweeney TE, Morton JM. Metabolic surgery: action via hormonal milieu changes, changes in bile acids or gut microbiome? A summary of the literature. Best Pract Res Clin Gastroenterol 2014;28(4):727–40.

24. Schauer PR, Bhatt DL, Kirwan JP, et al, STAMPEDE Investigators. Bariatric surgery versus intensive medical therapy for diabetes: 3-year outcomes. N Engl J Med 2014;370(21):2002–13.

25. Courcoulas AP, Belle SH, Neiberg RH, et al. Three-Year Outcomes of Bariatric Surgery vs Lifestyle Intervention for Type 2 Diabetes Mellitus Treatment: A Randomized Clinical Trial. JAMA Surg 2015;150(10):931–40.

26. Sjöström L. Review of the key results from the Swedish Obese Subjects (SOS) trial - a prospective controlled intervention study of bariatric surgery. J Intern Med 2013;273(3):219–34.

27. Puzziferri N, Roshek TB III, Mayo HG, et al. Long-term follow-up after bariatric surgery: a systematic review. JAMA 2014;312(9):934–42.

28. Chang SH, Stoll CR, Song J, et al. The effectiveness and risks of bariatric surgery: an updated systematic review and meta-analysis, 2003-2012. JAMA Surg 2014; 149(3):275–87.

29. Angrisani L, Santonicola A, Iovino P, et al. Bariatric surgery worldwide 2013. Obes Surg 2015;25:1822–32.

30. Chandarana K, Batterham RL. Shedding pounds after going under the knife: metabolic insights from cutting the gut. Nat Med 2012;18(5):668–9.
31. Papamargaritis D, le Roux CW, Sioka E, et al. Changes in gut hormone profile and glucose homeostasis after laparoscopic sleeve gastrectomy. Surg Obes Relat Dis 2013;9(2):192–201.
32. Herron DM, Roohipour R. Bariatric surgical anatomy and mechanisms of action. Gastrointest Endosc Clin N Am 2011;21(2):213–28.
33. Arterburn D, Johnson ES, Butler MG, et al. Predicting 90-day mortality after bariatric surgery: an independent, external validation of the OS-MRS prognostic risk score. Surg Obes Relat Dis 2014;10(5):774–9.
34. Robinson AH, Adler S, Stevens HB, et al. What variables are associated with successful weight loss outcomes for bariatric surgery after 1 year? Surg Obes Relat Dis 2014;10(4):697–704.

Behavioral Modification for the Management of Obesity

Claire P. Kelley, PsyD[a],*, Geena Sbrocco, MS, RD[b,c],
Tracy Sbrocco, PhD[a]

KEYWORDS

- Obesity • Behavioral modification • Cognitive behavioral interventions for weight loss
- Weight management

KEY POINTS

- An understanding of and appreciation for the multifactorial and ecological nature of the etiology of obesity are important.
- There are significant obesity-related health disparities, particularly in African American women.
- Providing a nonstigmatizing approach to overweight and obese patients is important.
- Motivational interviewing techniques are effective within the patient-centered medical home; behaviorally based programs for obesity management inform patients of reasonable goals and expectations.
- Collaborating with behavioral health care specialists and registered dietitians also facilitate success as part of an integrated patient-centered approach to weight management.

INTRODUCTION: NATURE OF THE PROBLEM
Placing the Behavioral Management of Obesity in the Larger Context

In 2003, the US Preventive Services Task Force recommended that primary care practitioners (PCPs) screen all adults for obesity and offer behavioral interventions and intensive counseling for those identified as being obese.[1] This recommendation came at a time when fewer than half of primary care physicians were routinely discussing weight management with their patients.[2] In addition, there were no established evidence-based guidelines for behavioral weight loss counseling in primary care

The authors had been funded by NIH (P20MD000505); NIHMS-ID: 729321.
[a] Department of Medical and Clinical Psychology, Uniformed Services University of the Health Sciences, 4301 Jones Bridge Road, Bethesda, MD 20814-4799, USA; [b] Loyola University Chicago, Marcella Niehoff School of Nursing, 2160 South 1st Avenue, Maywood, IL 60153-3328, USA; [c] Lincoln Park Care Center, 499 Pine Brook Road, Lincoln Park, NJ 07035-1804, USA
* Corresponding author. Department of Medical and Clinical Psychology, Uniformed Services University of the Health Sciences, 4301 Jones Bridge Road, B1022-B, Bethesda, MD 20814-4799.
E-mail address: claire.kelley.ctr@usuhs.edu

Prim Care Clin Office Pract 43 (2016) 159–175
http://dx.doi.org/10.1016/j.pop.2015.10.004
0095-4543/16/$ – see front matter © 2016 Elsevier Inc. All rights reserved.

settings.[3] Obesity is a complex combination of genetic, biological, psychological, and sociocultural factors. Health behaviors such as eating patterns and volitional physical activity are under the complex influence of many psychological and social factors.[4] Viewing obesity in the context of a complex interaction between genetics and environment guides the understanding of the condition and helps form multidimensional treatment plans. Addressing the social and psychological cues associated with overeating and low physical activity through behavioral modification helps patients see success in the context of individual weight management goals.[5–7]

This article provides primary care–based behavioral strategies for working with obese patients and their families. A multifactorial model for obesity is presented. Strategies for creating effective patient encounters and specific recommendations to motivate and support patients are provided. Multicomponent programs include nutritional, physical activity, and cognitive behavioral approaches to target overweight/obesity. This article focuses on behavioral strategies for weight management.

Weight Stigma

The discussion of the behavioral management of obesity must include an understanding of weight stigma. Overweight is often stigmatized in American culture. This, unfortunately, includes health care providers.[8] Individual provider biases must be recognized and overcome to develop treatment environments that welcome overweight and obese patients (**Boxes 1** and **2**). Providers often view obese patients as lazy, weak-willed, and noncompliant.[9] Patients perceive these biases and delay or avoid seeking care because they anticipate being disrespected.[10,11] As a result, obese patients are *less* likely to obtain recommended preventive health services. Obese patients are also more likely to cancel appointments or delay care,[12–14] which creates an unhealthy paradox whereby patients requiring medical care actively avoid it. Health care providers should use language appropriately when referring to patients with overweight/obesity, actively avoiding stigmatizing words or phrases (**Box 3**).[15]

An Ecological Model for Understanding Obesity: Understanding Microsystem and Macrosystem Factors to Produce Change

Environmental factors that determine an individual's weight-related health behaviors occur at the *microsystem level* (family/social determinants) and *macrosystem level* (eg, cultural and social values).[16] Some of these are modifiable and others are not. This microsystem/macrosystem concept aligns well with the modern patient-centered medical home (PCMH) model of health care. The PCMH emphasizes caring for the patient in the context of his or her "unique needs, culture, values, and preferences."[17]

Macrosystem factors promoting obesity include the marketing of calorie-dense processed foods to certain segments of the population at increased risk for obesity. For example, African Americans view 50% more fast food television advertisements and dine more frequently at fast food restaurants than Caucasians.[18] Obesity-related

---

Box 1
Patient perspectives: weight stigma

I think the worst was my family doctor who made a habit of shrugging off my health concerns...The last time I went to him with a problem, he said, "You just need to learn to push yourself away from the table."

Box 2
Weight stigma: what you can do?

1. Realize obesity is a health problem, not an issue of personal appearance
2. Talk to patients about their current health status and goals
   a. Weight and BMI
   b. Laboratory values
   c. How they feel, in general
3. Make office accommodations for larger patients (eg, waiting room chairs, scales, examination tables)
4. Educate office/clinic staff about the importance of making overweight individuals feel welcome and not embarrassed

health disparities among African American individuals are discussed in more detail throughout this chapter.

Microsystem factors include how culture, family environment, and social settings impact eating and activity patterns (**Box 4**). For example, fewer food rules about where and when food may be eaten in the home are associated with increased weight.[19] Small changes to the household environment supports behavioral weight loss interventions (eg, no food allowed in front of television, avoid excessive snacking between meals). Families should be encouraged to work together to engage in healthy behaviors rather than just focusing on one person within the family who is struggling with weight (Tracy Sbrocco, PhD, unpublished data).[20]

Microsystem factors also involve issues relating to stimulus control. Environmental cues associated with overeating can be altered to assist weight loss and long-term weight maintenance. Patients and physicians should collaborate to identify individual stimuli that patients can avoid. Examples include eliminating television within the eating environment, removing snack foods from the home, and using smaller plates for meal consumption.[21]

Food intake is higher when individuals are distracted during meals.[22] Food consumption is associated with the length of the meal and the number of individuals at the table.[22,23] Individuals are less attentive to caloric intake when eating with company or while watching television. These distractions reduce the ability to self-monitor food consumption and can promote unintended weight gain.

Emotional eating also plays an important role in the management of overweight and obesity. Stress is a primary predictor of overeating and poor weight maintenance.[21]

Box 3
Patient-preferred terms

- Weight problem
- BMI
- Excess weight

Avoid the following:

- Fatness/Excess fat/Fat
- Obesity
- Large size
- Heavy

Box 4
Healthier environment: what can you do?

1. Encourage household rules to limit consumption of excess calories

2. Remove less healthy foods from the home

3. Limit mindless snacking

4. Restrict TV and video game time

5. Address family views on weight

6. Encourage stress management:
   a. Breathing exercises
   b. Progressive muscle relaxation
   c. Meditation

For information on stress management, see https://nccih.nih.gov/health/stress/relaxation.htm.

Acute and chronic stress alters the desire for food and subsequent food intake. Stress influences central reward pathways, resulting in consumption of higher calorie foods. Stress causes overeating, and stress is often suppressed by eating.[24] Patients must learn alternative methods for coping with stress (eg, diaphragmatic breathing, progressive muscle relaxation, mediation) to prevent stressed-induced overeating.

Cultural Competency in the Behavioral Management of Obesity

Not all cultures view overweight/obesity as a problem. This perspective relates to beauty ideals about ideal body size or health beliefs suggesting that bigger is healthier. Food-scarce environments are also obesogenic. For example, African American women (who are at particularly high risk for obesity) may be less likely to engage in traditional weight management programs and may experience decreased success when they do participate (**Box 5**).[25–27] Rather than "blame the victim," providers should work to engage these women and their families. African American women often have leadership roles in their families and are very influential in their children's eating patterns.[28] Engaging patients to provide culturally appropriate education and community-specific recommendations for change can have a broad impact.

Key points:
1. Obesity occurs in a large ecological context and is multifactorial in nature.
2. Many ecological and environmental factors contribute to and maintain overweight and obesity. Understanding these factors helps destigmatize obesity and promotes culturally appropriate treatment.

Box 5
Patient perspective: African American women

We really don't know a lot about healthiness [in eating]. Traditionally, most of our habits have been handed down to us. You eat all of the food on your plate and you have all this fat and that fat and more fat on top of fat…we really have a lack of knowledge when it comes to that and we learn it the hard way. You get sick…You've been taught this stuff all your life, but you never knew it was wrong.

BEHAVIORAL MODIFICATION FOR OBESITY MANAGEMENT
Treatment Basics

The behavioral treatment of obesity is noninvasive and relatively low cost. Behavioral interventions to promote lifestyle changes should include face-to-face contact and provide at least 14 sessions within the first 6 months to yield the best results.[29] These interventions are often conducted in group settings and may be available at local hospitals, through commercial programs or in the office setting. Behavioral interventions require time and commitment on the part of the patient and the provider. Patients can be referred to commercial or medical center–based behavioral group programs for weight loss and weight maintenance. If providing an outside referral, it is important that primary care physicians continue to provide ongoing support. Several simple behavioral principles[30,31] can easily be integrated into an office practice, as follows.

Collaborative goal setting
Setting reasonable goals that are achievable promotes long-term success. Patients often think they need to lose a great deal of weight to be successful. Helping patients choose a long-term weight loss goal that is reasonable and achievable (eg, 5% weight loss) increases the likelihood of successful adherence. Establish a specific goal for physical activity. Set a specific goal for dietary intake. Set a specific goal for weight management. When possible, tie other health outcomes (better blood pressure control, improved lipid profile) to the weight management goal to increase motivation and adherence.

Accountability
Incorporate a measure of accountability to each of the goals. How often will patients come into the office to assess weight-related goals? Have them participate in a program that meets weekly for several months with required sign-in. Which patients would succeed with an online program? Link established goals to office visits to assess progress and provide ongoing support and encouragement.

Nutrition consultation and meal planning
Having a registered dietitian nutritionist (RDN) visit with each patient and assess their knowledge and preferences also augments success. RDN expertise allows each patient to develop an individual nutrition plan that is culturally appropriate, practical, affordable, and achievable. When meeting with an RDN, a patient might expect to aim for the following:

- A daily reduction in caloric intake by 500 kilocalories (1200–1500 calories/d for women, 1500–1800 calories/d for men);
- An increase in physical activity to achieve 150 minutes per week of aerobic activity;
- Review of the Mifflin-St Jeor equation (recommended by the Academy of Nutrition and Dietetics to calculate metabolic rate [in kcal/d] in overweight or obese adults using actual body weight): multiply patient's resting energy expenditure by an activity factor to estimate needs. Energy needs should then be reduced by 500 to 750 kilocalories (3500–5250 kcal per week) for weight loss of 1 to 1.5 lb per week.[29,32]

Self-monitoring food intake, weight, and activity
Self-monitoring is the cornerstone of successful behavior therapy (**Boxes 6** and **7**). Monitoring food intake and activity levels directly increases self-awareness of personal behaviors. Self-monitoring slows down the decision-making process, allowing

---

Box 6
Patient perspective: I was a sloth!

It seems the older I got, the heavier I got. The weight just kept creeping up. It wasn't until my physician suggested I wear an activity monitor that I realized what a sloth I had become! My typical day involved only 2500 steps! I couldn't believe it at first. I went from my car, to the elevator, to my office, and back home. I now have a daily goal of 10,000 steps, which I usually make. I get up every hour and walk a quarter mile loop twice. It really adds up, I've lost weight, and I feel better!

---

individuals time to make healthier choices. Self-monitoring also alerts individuals about overconsumption and the nutritional content of foods.

- Smart phone applications allow patients to search for healthy food choices and record activities at little or no cost. Such applications allow for short- and long-term monitoring and augment weight loss treatment within primary care.[33] Examples include the following:
  - Goal setting for certain number of steps (10,000/d)
  - Prompts to get up and move after sedentary periods

Stimulus control

Stimulus control strategies alter an individual's environment to maximize healthy choices. An example is moving less healthy foods (or foods an individual tends to overeat) out of the house to limit consumption. A reminder note on the refrigerator or a prompt to exercise on the bathroom mirror are other examples of how to alter the home environment to promote healthy eating and exercise patterns.

Problem solving

Specific problem-solving tactics help patients explore their weight-related health behaviors. Using a behavioral chain to consider outcomes associated with different choices, patients are encouraged to consider different solutions before selecting the healthiest solution. Patients develop and implement a specific plan for the desired behavior and then evaluate the success of their solution. Patients are encouraged to think about problems differently and engage in creative problem solving. Group visits offer an ideal way to engage in problem solving that focuses on a specific health topic. Individuals learn from how others have handled similar problems and often create innovative solutions specific to their own circumstances.

Box 7
Patient perspective: I ate what?

My nutritionist had me record the food I was eating before I tried to lose any weight. She wanted me to understand the kinds of foods I was eating and where I might "get into trouble" as I try a new way of eating. It was such an eye opener! I just could NOT believe there were almost 200 calories in ½ cup of macaroni and cheese. And, let me tell you, a ½ cup was not my serving size—I was eating 2 ½ cups! Yes, that's almost 900 calories. I still eat it, but now I know to be sure to watch my portion sizes and not eat it as often if I want to maintain my weight loss.

Problem solving: troubleshooting specific eating situations
Social eating and eating outside of the home Restaurants are a potential bonanza for excessive caloric intake. Patients must learn skills for healthy eating outside of the home (**Box 8**). Americans eat more meals outside of the home than ever before. Dining out is no longer a rare event and, as such, cannot be used as an excuse for overeating. Controlling social eating and caloric consumption outside of the home must include an understanding of the impact this type of eating has on an individual's weight. The challenges of dining out include portion size, type of food, food preparation techniques, and the desire or habit of eating everything on the plate.

Emotional eating Many people eat in response to a variety of emotions, including anger, boredom, stress, anxiety, and frustration. Such eating behaviors have a significant influence on weight or health (**Box 9**).

Relapse prevention
Slip-ups are normal when initiating any lifestyle changes (**Box 10**). Learning how to get back on track is important. Necessary components of relapse prevention include the following:

- Understand the social cues that relate to both healthy and unhealthy weight-related behaviors. Patients should generate strategies to help navigate social events, travel, and vacations that commonly challenge the ability to make healthy lifestyle choices.
- Stress management is essential. Patients should be encouraged to use a variety of techniques including problem solving, regular physical activity, relaxation

---

Box 8
Tips for eating out

1. Do NOT skip meals before eating out. Being hungry makes it more difficult to think and plan wisely.

2. Plan ahead. Choose a restaurant that has a wide variety of choices.

3. There are new rules for buffets! Do not overfill your plate. Choose a little bit. Cut back on portions. Make one pass and call it quits.

4. *Study the menu* carefully. Order items that are broiled, baked, poached, or steamed. Limit fried, buttered, or creamed foods, or items with sauce/gravy.

5. *Ask questions* about the food before you place an order. Inquire about preparation methods.

6. Ask for dressing, sauce and gravy *on the side*.

7. Fresh rolls or breads are delicious without added butter.

8. *Portion sizes.* Consider the following strategies to limit portion sizes:
   - Split a meal or item with someone.
   - Order à la carte (side dishes or appetizers).

9. Decide what you are going to eat before you dig in. Put the remainder to the side. Take it home.

10. Use *alcohol* sparingly.

11. *Salad bars.* People think of salads as "free food." They are not. Dressing, bacon, high-fat cheeses, and premixed salads are high in calories.

12. Beware of *eating on the run!* Fast food restaurant choices tend to be abundant in fat and calories. Take lower fat food choices with you.

Box 9
Where does emotional eating come from?

Our culture often takes care of its people with food. Children who are upset might be offered a lollipop or an ice cream cone. Parents often soothe children with food. Food comes to be associated with comfort.

It is important to help patients and families find other ways to deal with negative feelings.

Box 10
Sample dialogue for helping patients understand and plan for slips and prevent relapses

Slips

A slip is an error. You did something you really did not want to do. A slip stops there. Say, for example, you intended to enjoy one cookie and wound up eating 10. If you can see this as temporary, spend a bit of time trying to figure out how you did this and make sure to treat it as a Learning Experience rather than a failure, you'll be okay.

In the big picture, 10 cookies are not going to make you overweight or keep you overweight. However, if you let one slip turn into a series of slips, you are on the road to Relapse. Again, it is your belief about what you've done that causes you trouble, not what actually happened. Know the difference between a Learning Experience and a Failure. A failure attitude does not lead to success. Learning, on the other hand, is a lifelong endeavor.

Physical activity example: planning for an exercise slip

The time changes; seasons change, or you get bored or injured. All of these are common reasons that call for a change in an exercise routine. Rather than denying that this could ever happen to you, look ahead and anticipate what can cause you problems. Anticipate and plan. For each potential problem, what will you do?

---

exercises, engaging social supports, or other cognitive strategies (eg, positive self-talk).
- Maintaining motivation over the long term can be a challenge. Acknowledge personal successes, engage in regular review of progress, reassess goals, and set new goals as necessary. Primary care physicians are well-positioned to help patients with weight management over the long term.

Box 11 summarizes effective behavioral strategies for weight loss.

Box 11
Effective behavioral strategies for weight loss

- Self-monitoring of nutritional intake and physical activity
- Goal setting
- Problem solving
- Social support
- Stress management
- Stimulus control
- Alternative behaviors (identifying internal cues for eating, such as craving and finding alternate behaviors rather than giving in to the craving)

- Cognitive restructuring
- Contingency management—making specific plans for slip-ups
- Continuous care—the value of a patient-centered medical home
- Establish a weight management range
- Construct a weight maintenance plan
- Meet with an RDN to discuss structured meal plans, meal replacements, and understanding of portion sizes and portion control
- Develop specific relapse prevention techniques[32,34]

RESEARCH REVIEW: PROTOTYPICAL PROGRAMS FOR BEHAVIORAL MODIFICATION IN THE MANAGEMENT OF OBESITY

Archetypal weight loss research studies such as the Diabetes Prevention Program (DPP) and the Look AHEAD (Action for Health in Diabetes) trial (based on the DPP but administered in a group setting) provide valuable information on eating patterns and physical activity habits that are associated with weight loss. They also highlight behavioral strategies as the hallmarks of a successful cognitive behavioral weight loss intervention to help in weight loss efforts. The DPP program has proven efficacy in a primary care setting, using either coaches or a home-based DVD approach.[35] These trials have resulted in long-term weight loss after 10 years and longer delay in onset of diabetes in the lifestyle intervention group (as compared with the placebo and the metformin medication group).[6] Weight loss among those in the lifestyle intervention was approximately 5% of body weight, whereas those in the usual care condition of diabetes support and education lost only 2% of body weight.[7] Overall, half of the lifestyle intervention participants lost more than 5% of their body weight[7] and decreased risk factors for cardiovascular disease.[36] Over a quarter of these participants lost 10% of their body weight or more.[7]

CHANGING LIFESTYLES FOR LONG-TERM WEIGHT MANAGEMENT: BACKGROUND ON NONDIETING BEHAVIORAL MODIFICATION APPROACHES

Although studies such as the Look AHEAD and DPP trials boast low attrition rates (94% retention in the Look AHEAD randomized cohort[7] and 98% retention in the randomized cohort of the DPP[5]), these interventions require substantial calorie deficit (eg, cutting at least 500 calories per day from intake). Behavioral weight loss interventions have yielded significant results in adherent participants, but many studies report high attrition rates (up to 50% in those emphasizing food intake restriction). These studies also show that patients have significant difficulty maintaining weight loss, exhibit marked after-intervention weight regain,[37] and also show potentially negative psychological impacts (eg, attributing self-worth with weight loss success) associated with dieting.[38,39] The self-discipline required to be successful in these weight loss programs often requires adhering to a strict diet and may engender a pattern of restraint that paradoxically leads to compensatory overeating.[40] Diet-approach interventions are sometimes followed by a pattern of slow weight regain that results in participants returning to baseline weight.[41]

A FEASIBLE ALTERNATIVE: FEATURES OF NONDIET APPROACHES TO WEIGHT MANAGEMENT

Recent obesity research focuses on a nondiet approach due to difficulty adhering to low-calorie diets over the long term. The nondieting approach shifts the focus from weight loss to improvements in overall health.[42] Small, manageable changes and a healthy lifestyle are emphasized rather than a sole focus on weight loss/control.[40] Moderation leads to a balanced approach to eating and exercise.[41] Goals include steady weight loss and maintenance of lost weight as well as overall physical and psychological well-being. Nondiet strategies also appear to offer some protection against disordered eating behaviors (eg, food restriction and binge eating).[43] Nondiet interventions have lower attrition rates and longer-term adherence because participants are more able to follow realistic eating plans.[38] Intuitive eating and behavioral choice treatment (BCT) are examples of nondieting approaches. These are promising approaches and an overview of these modalities follows. However, a caveat is that these results from studies using nondieting methods may not be fully supportive. As an example, some studies showed negligible or clinically insignificant weight loss.[38,44]

Intuitive Eating

Intuitive eating includes an unrestricted permission to eat. Intuitive eating allows individuals to eat for physical reasons as opposed to emotional reasons. This technique teaches patients to focus on internal hunger and satiety cues to guide food consumption and also emphasizes body-food choice congruence.[42] Intuitive eating is associated with improvements in body mass index (BMI) and healthy weight maintenance, improved long-term weight maintenance, and decreased unhealthy diet behaviors (caloric restriction and binge eating).[42,45]

Nondieting Approach: Behavioral Choice Treatment

BCT is an example of a weight management program that de-emphasizes significant caloric restriction and aims for moderation in healthy eating and exercise patterns. It is typically a group-based intervention. Participants are taught to view eating and exercise as choices. When healthy weight–related behavior choices are made, permanent weight and health changes are likely to follow. Significant emphasis is placed on how participant choices are linked to weight outcomes, regulation of hunger, and a general feeling of well-being. BCT includes individual exploration of previous negative outcomes following poor food or exercise choices (eg, regret after indulging in "bad foods"). Cognitive restructuring is introduced as a tool to prevent these negative outcomes. Steady weight loss is set as a realistic expectation of the program. BCT emphasizes that there are no forbidden foods. Participants learn to recognize high-calorie, high-carbohydrate, or high-fat food choices and moderate consumption accordingly. Participants maintain a weekly food diary and engage in a moderate program of physical activity, starting with 15 minutes of walking per day 3 times per week with the ultimate target of walking 180 minutes each week. The key skills of BCT include moderating caloric restriction through small changes in eating and exercise. Patients learn self-monitoring, are encouraged to engage social support networks, and augment self-efficacy to sustain behaviors over time.[46]

RESEARCH REVIEW: BEHAVIORAL CHOICE TREATMENT

Disparately higher rates of obesity are found among African American women,[47] thus interventions addressing this health disparity could potentially impact national obesity rates. BCT has yielded a steady, measured reduction in weight over time (12 and 24 months), whereas traditional behavior therapy participants (adhering to the typical restraint model for dieting to include reduced caloric intake, self-monitoring, stimulus control, and behavioral substitution) have regained lost weight.[48] BCT and its offshoot, behavioral choice treatment with a family component (BCTF) that adds a family module, has been used successfully over the last decade and a half in research and community settings with Caucasian and African American individuals (Tracy Sbrocco, PhD, unpublished data).[48–53]

PRIMARY CARE PLAN OF ACTION: FRAMEWORK FOR BUILDING A CLINICAL PROGRAM IN THE BEHAVIORAL MODIFICATION IN THE MANAGEMENT OF OBESITY

Programs implemented in clinical settings contrast with research intervention trials. Behavioral health specialists with expertise in weight management, therefore, are ideal collaborators to help their obese patients succeed in weight loss. Improved adherence, increased motivation for attending more sessions, and an emphasis on more intensive and longer-term treatment are important elements of success.[54] Low-intensity (less than 2 visits per month) physician counseling is not likely to yield the same results as intense counseling (at least 2 visits per month for the first 3 months).[55]

Spotlight on: motivating overweight/obese veterans everywhere! a veteran's administration medical center weight management program

- *MOVE!* (Motivating Overweight/Obese Veterans Everywhere) is an evidence-based intervention that has been utilized nation-wide since 2006[56] and serves as an example of a widely disseminated behavioral modification program for the management of obesity with an interdisciplinary collaborative focus.

- Incorporates a person-centered individualized and group-support approach to obesity that includes many of the cognitive and behavioral treatment components discussed above (e.g., self-monitoring, goal setting, stimulus control).[56,57]

- Intended to be easily implemented as a part of each veteran's care via their primary care clinic.[56]

- For further study… http://www.move.va.gov/

Results show that….

- Moderate weight loss has been noted in these programs over short term follow up periods (e.g., up through 12 months post-intervention participation).[58] Though veterans participating in an intense and sustained delivery of the *MOVE!* program experience some short term weight loss, the average number of *MOVE!* visits is less than 5 (in 2010) and more than half of *MOVE!* patients have only two visits or less per year.[54]

A COLLABORATIVE APPROACH: PRIMARY CARE PHYSICIANS AND BEHAVIORAL HEALTH SPECIALISTS

Primary care physicians collaborating with behavioral health specialists have the distinct opportunity to facilitate patients' motivation for weight loss. Increased patient motivation leads to increased adherence and improves the likelihood of success. Two practical primary care techniques to facilitate patient motivation include (1) motivational interviewing (MI) and (2) BCTF—a family-based approach to the behavioral modification in the management of obesity.

Motivational Interviewing

Primary care physicians are often the first health care provider with whom patients discuss weight loss goals. This office visit with the primary care physician is an excellent opportunity to have a meaningful and motivating conversation about patient-specific goals. MI is a therapeutic modality that has its origins in counseling for alcohol abuse.[59] MI has been used for behavior change in obesity[60] and many other health conditions. MI is a person-centered, goal-directed approach that augments an individual patient's intrinsic motivation for committing to behavior change. Working with and through a patient's ambivalence to elicit behavior change is a hallmark of MI.[61] MI aligns well with weight management objectives by eliciting behavior change within the context of a positive provider-patient relationship.

MI is a patient-centered approach with the following core principles:

- Express empathy
- Support the patient's self-efficacy
- Roll with resistance
- Develop discrepancy[61]

Empathic and reflective listening is central to MI. The acronym OARS describes core elements of MI:

- O: ask open questions
- A: affirm the patient's perspective
- R: reflect what was heard to ensure understanding
- S: summarize shared understanding to set specific goals[61]

Tips for Motivational Interviewing

1. Determine the patient's desire for change: "On a scale of 1 to 10, how important is achieving a healthy weight status as a goal for you?"
2. Determine patient confidence in their ability to make the change: "On a scale of 1 to 10, how confident are you that you can make the necessary changes to achieve a healthy weight status?"
3. Obtain a commitment (verbally or, preferably, in writing) to making the necessary changes.[61]
4. Do not oppose a patient if they are resistant to change ("roll with resistance").
5. Summarize the patient's "change talk" as part of a patient-centered dialogue.
6. Create a patient-directed plan for making necessary changes.[61]
7. Understand that motivational interviewing principles are a part of a comprehensive behavioral weight management program.[61]
8. Appreciate how the principles of motivational interviewing integrate well within the PCMH model of care.[62]

RESEARCH REVIEW: MOTIVATIONAL INTERVIEWING

In a review of randomized controlled trials using MI for weight loss among overweight/obese individuals, medium effect sizes were found for the reduction of body mass compared with a control intervention.[60] MI is effective in helping patients make dietary and physical activity changes to manage diabetes,[63] which has implications in the management of obesity. MI techniques are easily learned within a reasonable time commitment and yield positive results relevant to obesity-related conditions.[64] Over one-third of MI interventions for obesity in primary care settings showed significant weight loss compared with a control condition.[65]

BEHAVIORAL CHOICE TREATMENT WITH A FAMILY COMPONENT

Because of the alarming rates of obesity in the United States, particularly among non-Hispanic black and Hispanic youth and adults, there is a clear need to understand the manner in which the family environment influences obesity. Little research focuses on family interventions for weight loss, and studies with diverse samples are scarce.[66]

Thus, a family-based approach to behavioral modification for obesity management likely offers a solution that fits the problem. A family-based approach focusing on an entire family's weight-related health behaviors is a novel primary care intervention.

Previous success in weight loss in both Caucasian and African American participants has been demonstrated with BCT.[48,52] A planned collaboration between primary care physicians and behavioral health specialists using the BCTF approach addresses obesity across many ethnic groups. Treatment approaches that consider the ecological context and environment of the patient conceptualize obesity from a more comprehensive perspective. The BCTF program harnesses the impact of positive changes in the household environment and engages families to promote healthy weight loss efforts.[20,66,67]

Target participants (primary participants) in BCTF engage in a behavioral weight management program with family members (secondary participants) and have their progress assessed throughout the intervention.[68] A family module is included with each topic. Primary participants are provided with family meal plans and handouts on healthy snacks and drinks for children and family, and tips for healthy and quick-packed lunches. Verbal encouragement is used to motivate participants during group sessions. Primary participants are encouraged to set family goals in addition to their individual weight loss/health goals (eg, whole family physical activity sessions, increased fruit and vegetable consumption, and limiting fast food dinners).

The BCTF treatment model serves as one example of a behavioral modification approach to the management of obesity that is appropriately administered in a primary care setting. Understanding the basic principles of cognitive behavioral therapy and MI allows primary care physicians to create a holistic partnership with patients and families to work together toward weight management goals.

Spotlight on obesity health disparities: behavioral choice treatment and behavioral choice treatment with a family component research in African American women

BCT interventions within community settings have demonstrated success in improved weight loss outcomes among African American individuals.[49–52] A recent trial run of BCTF in a community setting with African American women indicates weight loss among both primary participants and their family members. Although there was some tendency toward regain of some of the lost weight at after-intervention follow-up time points, participants lost weight overall when assessed at the 12-month follow-up session (Tracy Sbrocco, PhD, unpublished data).

Key points:
1. MI techniques translate well in the PCMH setting.
2. A sample behavioral modification weight loss program with a family focus serves as a potential interdisciplinary model for weight management.

SUMMARY

An interdisciplinary, PCMH approach to weight management in primary care settings includes multiple factors. An understanding of and appreciation for the multifactorial and ecological nature of the cause of obesity is important. There are significant obesity-related health disparities, particularly in African American women. Providing a nonstigmatizing approach to overweight and obese patients is important. MI techniques are effective within the PCMH. Behaviorally based programs for obesity management inform patients of reasonable goals and expectations.[69] Collaborating with behavioral health care specialists and registered dietitians also facilitates success as part of an integrated patient-centered approach to weight management.

DISCLAIMER

The opinions expressed herein are those of the authors and are not necessarily representative of those of the Uniformed Services University or the Department of Defense.

FUNDING/SUPPORT

This work was supported in part by Award Number P20 MD000505 from the National Institute on Minority Health and Health Disparities. The content is solely the responsibility of the authors and does not necessarily represent the official views of the National Institute on Minority Health and Health Disparities or the National Institutes of Health.

REFERENCES

1. Preventive Services Task Force. Screening for obesity in adults: recommendations and rationale. Ann Intern Med 2003;139:930–2.
2. Simkin-Silverman LR, Conroy MB, King WC, et al. Treatment of overweight and obesity in primary care practice: current evidence and future directions. Am J Lifestyle Med 2008;2(4):296–304.
3. Wadden TA, Volger S, Tsai AG, et al. Managing obesity in primary care practice: an overview with perspective from the POWER-UP study. Int J Obes 2005;37(S1):S3–11.
4. World Health Organization. Obesity and Overweight Fact Sheet. 2015. Available at: http://www.who.int/mediacentre/factsheets/fs311/en/. Accessed June 4, 2015.
5. Diabetes Prevention Program Research Group. First versus repeat treatment with a lifestyle intervention program: attendance and weight loss outcomes. Int J Obes 2008;32:1537–44.
6. Diabetes Prevention Program Research Group. 10-year follow-up of diabetes incidence and weight loss in the Diabetes Prevention Program Outcomes Study. Lancet 2009;374(9702):1677–86.
7. Look AHEAD Research Group. Eight-year weight losses with an intensive lifestyle intervention: the Look AHEAD Study. Obesity (Silver Spring) 2014;22(1):5–13.
8. Puhl RM, Heuer CA. The stigma of obesity: a review and update. Obesity (Silver Spring) 2009;17:941–64.
9. Puhl RM, Brownell KD. Confronting and coping with weight stigma: an investigation of overweight and obese adults. Obesity (Silver Spring) 2006;14(10):1802–15.
10. Bertakis KD, Azari R. The impact of obesity on primary care visits. Obes Res 2005;13(9):1615–23.
11. Edmunds L. Parents' perceptions of health professionals' responses when seeking help for their overweight children. Fam Pract 2005;22:287–92.
12. Drury CA, Louis M. Exploring the association between body weight, stigma of obesity, and health care avoidance. J Am Acad Nurse Pract 2002;14(12):554–61.
13. Olson CL, Schumaker HD, Yawn BP. Overweight women delay medical care. Arch Fam Med 1994;3(10):888–92.
14. Jones K. Weight stigma among providers decreases the quality of care received by obese patients. Hillsboro (OR): School of Physician Assistant Studies; 2010. Paper 207.

15. Volger S, Vetter ML, Dougherty M, et al. Patients' preferred terms for describing their excess weight: discussing obesity in clinical practice. Obesity (Silver Spring) 2012;20(1):147–50.

16. Brofenbrenner U. Ecological models of human development. In: Gauvain M, Cole M, editors. International Encylopedia of Education, Vol 3, 2nd Ed. Oxford: Elsvier Reprinted. Readings on the Development of Children, 2nd Ed. New York: Freeman; 1993. p. 37–43.

17. United States Department of Health and Human Services. Defining the Patient Centered Medical Home. 2015. Available at: http://www.pcmh.ahrq.gov/page/defining-pcmh. Accessed May 13, 2015.

18. Williams JD, Crockett D, Harrison RL, et al. The role of food culture and marketing activity in health disparities. Prev Med 2012;55(5):382–6.

19. Thomas JL, Stewart DW, Lynam IM, et al. Support needs of overweight African American women for weight loss. Am J Health Behav 2009;33(4):339–52.

20. Gorin AA, Raynor HA, Fava J, et al. Randomized controlled trial of a comprehensive home environment-focused weight-loss program for adults. Health Psychol 2013;32(2):128–37.

21. Kumanyika SK, Obarzanek E, Stettler N, et al. Population-based prevention of obesity: the need for comprehensive promotion of healthful eating, physical activity, and energy balance: a scientific statement from American Heart Association Council on Epidemiology and Prevention, Interdisciplinary Committee for Prevention (formerly the expert panel on population and prevention science). Circulation 2008;118(4):428–64.

22. Hetherington MM, Anderson AS, Norton GN, et al. Situational effects on meal intake: a comparison of eating alone and eating with others. Physiol Behav 2006;88(4):498–505.

23. Bell R, Pliner PL. Time to eat: the relationship between the number of people eating and meal duration in three lunch settings. Appetite 2003;41(2):215–8.

24. Sominsky L, Spencer SJ. Eating behavior and stress: a pathway to obesity. Front Psychol 2014;5:434.

25. McTigue KM, Harris R, Hemphill B, et al. Screening interventions for obesity in adults: summary of the evidence for the U.S. preventive services task force. Ann Intern Med 2003;139(11):933–49.

26. West DS, Prewitt ET, Bursac Z, et al. Weight loss of black, white, and Hispanic men and women in the Diabetes Prevention Program. Obesity (Silver Spring) 2008;16(6):1413–20.

27. Wing RR, Anglin K. Effectiveness of a behavioral weight control program for blacks and whites with NIDDM. Diabetes Care 1996;19(5):403–13.

28. Kumanyika SK, Whitt-Glover MC, Gary TL, et al. Expanding the obesity research paradigm to reach African American communities. Prev Chronic Dis 2007;4(4):A112.

29. American College of Cardiology, American Heart Association Task Force on Practice Guidelines, The Obesity Society. Executive summary: guidelines (2013) for the management of overweight and obesity in adults. Obesity (Silver Spring) 2013;22(Suppl 22):S5–39.

30. Diabetes Prevention Program Research Group. The Diabetes Prevention Program (DPP): description of lifestyle intervention. Diabetes Care 2002;25(12):2165–71.

31. Look AHEAD Research Group. Look AHEAD (Action for Health in Diabetes): design and methods for a clinical trial of weight loss for the prevention of cardiovascular disease in type 2 diabetes. Control Clin Trials 2003;24:610–28.

32. Academy of Nutrition and Dietetics. Adult weight management (AWM) Guideline. 2014. Available at: http://www.andeal.org/topic.cfm?menu=5276&cat=4688. Accessed June 27, 2015.

33. Spring B, Duncan JM, Janke EA, et al. Integrating technology into standard weight loss treatment: a randomized controlled trial. JAMA Intern Med 2013;173(2):105.

34. Grave RD, Centis E, Marzocchi R, et al. Major factors for facilitating change in behavioral strategies to reduce obesity. Psychol Res Behav Manag 2013;6:101–10.

35. Ma J, Yank V, Xiao L, et al. Translating the diabetes prevention program lifestyle intervention for weight loss into primary care: a randomized trial. JAMA Intern Med 2013;173(2):113–21.

36. Wing RR, Lang W, Wadden TA, et al. Benefits of modest weight loss in improving cardiovascular risk factors in overweight and obese individuals with type 2 diabetes. Diabetes Care 2011;34(7):1481–6.

37. Dansinger ML, Tatsioni A, Wong JB, et al. Meta-analysis: the effect of dietary counseling for weight loss. Ann Intern Med 2007;147(1):41–50.

38. Bacon L, Keim NL, VanLoan MD, et al. Evaluating a 'non-diet' wellness intervention for improvement of metabolic fitness, psychological well-being and eating and activity behaviors. Int J Obes Relat Metab Disord 2002;26(6):854–65.

39. Hession M, Rolland C, Kulkarni U, et al. Systematic review of randomized controlled trials of low-carbohydrate vs. low-fat/low-calorie diets in the management of obesity and its comorbidities. Obes Rev 2009;10:36–50.

40. Polivy J, Herman CP. Undieting: a program to help people stop dieting. Int J Eat Disord 1992;11:261–8.

41. Seagle HM, Strain GW, Makris A, et al. Position of the American Dietetic Association: weight management. J Am Diet Assoc 2009;109(2):330–46.

42. Schaefer JT, Magnuson AB. A review of interventions that promote eating by internal cues. J Acad Nutr Diet 2014;114(5):734–60.

43. Laliberte M, Newton M, McCabe R, et al. Controlling your weight versus controlling your lifestyle: how beliefs about weight control affect risk for disordered eating, body dissatisfaction and self-esteem. Cognit Ther Res 2007;31:852–69.

44. Wadden TA, Foster GD, Sarwer DB, et al. Dieting and the development of eating disorders in obese women: results of a randomized controlled trial. Am J Clin Nutr 2004;80(3):560.

45. Van Dyke N, Drinkwater EJ. Relationships between intuitive eating and health indicators: literature review. Public Health Nutr 2014;17(8):1757–66.

46. Sbrocco T. Behavior choice treatment manual. Bethesda (MD): Uniformed Services University of the Health Sciences; 1999.

47. Ogden CL, Carroll MD, Kit BK, et al. Prevalence of childhood and adult obesity in the United States, 2011-2012. J Am Med Assoc 2014;311(8):806–14.

48. Sbrocco T, Nedegaard RC, Stone JM, et al. Behavioral choice treatment promotes continuing weight loss: preliminary results of a cognitive behavioral decision-based treatment for obesity. J Consult Clin Psychol 1999;67:260–6.

49. Kennedy BM, Paeratakul S, Champagne CM, et al. A pilot church-based weight loss program for African-American adults using church members as health educators: a comparison of individual and group intervention. Ethn Dis 2005;15:373–8.

50. Kumanyika SK, Charleston JB. Lose weight and win: a church-based weight loss program for blood pressure control among black women. Patient Educ Couns 1992;19:19–32.

51. McNabb W, Quinn M, Kerver J, et al. The PATHWAYS church-based weight loss program for urban African-American women at risk for diabetes. Diabetes Care 1997;20:1518–23.

52. Sbrocco T, Carter MM, Lewis EL, et al. Church-based obesity treatment for African-American women improves adherence. Ethn Dis 2005;15:246–55.
53. Sbrocco T, Osborn R, Clark RD, et al. Assessing the stages of change among African American women in a weight management program. J Black Psychol 2011; 1(38):81–103.
54. Kahwati LC, Lance TX, Jones KR, et al. RE-AIM evaluation of the Veterans Health Administration's MOVE! Weight Management Program. Transl Behav Med 2011; 1(4):551–60.
55. Tsai AG, Wadden TA. Treatment of obesity in primary care practice in the United States: a systematic review. J Gen Intern Med 2009;24(9):1073–9.
56. Kinsinger LS, Jones KR, Kahwati L, et al. Design and dissemination of the MOVE! Weight-Management Program for Veterans. Prev Chronic Dis 2009;6(3):A98.
57. United States Department of Veterans Affairs. MOVE! Weight Management Program. (n.d.). Available at: http://www.move.va.gov/. Accessed August 17, 2015.
58. Dahn JR, Fitzpatrick SL, Llabre MM, et al. Weight management for Veterans: examining change in weight before and after MOVE! Obesity (Silver Spring) 2011;19(5):977–81.
59. Miller WR. Motivational interviewing with problem drinkers. Behavioural Psychotherapy 1983;11(2):147–72.
60. Armstrong MJ, Mottershead TA, Ronksley PE, et al. Motivational interviewing to improve weight loss in overweight and/or obese patients: a systematic review and meta-analysis of randomized controlled trials. Obes Rev 2011;12:709–23.
61. Miller WR, Rollnick S. Motivational interviewing: preparing people for change. New York: Guilford Press; 2002.
62. American Academy of Family Physicians, American College of Physicians, American Academy of Pediatrics, American Osteopathic Association. Joint Principles of the Patient Centered Medical Home. 2007. Available at: http://www.aafp.org/dam/AAFP/documents/practice_management/pcmh/initiatives/PCMHJoint.pdf. Accessed May 21, 2015.
63. Martins RK, McNeil DW. Review of motivational interviewing in promoting health behaviors. Clin Psychol Rev 2009;29:283–93.
64. Söderlund LL, Madson MB, Rubak S, et al. A systematic review of motivational interviewing training for general health care practitioners. Patient Educ Couns 2011;84(1):16–26.
65. Barnes RD, Ivejaz V. A systematic review of motivational interviewing for weight loss among adults in primary care. Obes Rev 2015;16:304–18.
66. Samuel-Hodge CD, Gizlice Z, Cai J, et al. Family functioning and weight loss in a sample of African Americans and whites. Ann Behav Med 2010;40:294–301.
67. Yanek LR, Becker DM, Moy TF, et al. Project joy: faith based cardiovascular health promotion for African American women. Public Health Rep 2001;116(Suppl 1): 68–81. Available at: http://www-ncbi-nlm-nih-gov.proxy.lib.odu.edu/pmc/articles/PMC1913665/pdf/pubhealthrep00206-0070.pdf. Accessed January 8, 2014.
68. Uniformed Services University of the Health Sciences Center for Health Disparities. Behavior choice treatment manual - family version. Bethesda (MD): Uniformed Services University of the Health Sciences; 2004.
69. American College of Physicians. Sample Care Coordination Agreement Referrals, Consults, Co- Management - General: for all patients. (n.d.). Available at: https://hvc.acponline.org/sample-care-coordination-agreement.pdf. Accessed June 10, 2015.

Printed and bound by CPI Group (UK) Ltd, Croydon, CR0 4YY

03/10/2024

01040487-0019